Make:
Bicycle Projects

John Baichtal

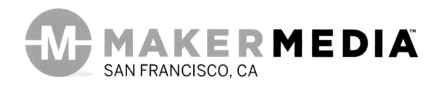

MAKER MEDIA
SAN FRANCISCO, CA

Make: Bicycle Projects

by John Baichtal

Printed in Canada.

Published by Maker Media, Inc., 1160 Battery Street East, Suite 125, San Francisco, CA 94111.

Maker Media books may be purchased for educational, business, or sales promotional use. Online editions are also available for most titles (*http://safaribooksonline.com*). For more information, contact our corporate/institutional sales department: 800-998-9938 or *corporate@oreilly.com*.

Editor: Patrick Di Justo	**Interior Designer:** David Futato
Production Editor: Melanie Yarbrough	**Cover Designer:** Sergio Burgos
Copyeditor: Jasmine Kwityn	**Cover Illustrations:** Adam Esat and Nate Van Dyke
Proofreader: Charles Roumeliotis	
Indexer: WordCo Indexing Services	**Illustrator:** Rebecca Demarest

August 2015:   First Edition

Revision History for the First Edition

2015-08-05:   First Release

See *http://oreilly.com/catalog/errata.csp?isbn=9781457186431* for release details.

978-1-457-18643-1

[TI]

Table of Contents

Preface

Nearly everything we own can't be modified, or requires the help of an expert. Some gearheads can fix their own cars but most of us can't. Techies can open up a computer and add or replace components, but many users are afraid to. What if you messed it up?

Bicycles are one of the few devices we own that not only are user modifiable, but most riders already have done so, if only by adding more air to the tires or adjusting the seat and handlebars. All but the least tool-savvy rider can easily add a beverage holder or horn, and kids apply stickers and other decorations all the time.

Perhaps price is a factor. You can get a decent used bike for $50 that will last you for years, but a similarly priced computer will be e-waste within a few months. If you were to wreck your bike trying to modify it, well, it's not like it was a $10,000 car. This lowers the fear factor and encourages adventuresome modifications.

That said, it's not all easy. Over the decades bike builders have settled on a rather complicated set of tools to loosen each part, and performing major mods necessitates having access to these tools. There is a learning curve as well, forcing you to research how to assemble gear cassettes and reconfigure chains.

And that's just the mechanical aspect. Makers have access to any number of resources for customizing their rides and making them work better. Electronics comes to mind—many bike riders have learned how to add sensors, microcontrollers, and other electronics to their bicycles.

A tiny subset practices the most radical of modifications: "frankensteining" two bikes together to form a new one, welding the tubes together themselves. Even more radically, some people simply weld up their own frames from steel tubing, to make it more truly their own.

I wrote *Make: Bicycle Projects* to encourage readers to make any and all of those modifications. If all you're comfortable with is creating your own bike basket or tightening a spoke, I got you covered. If you're ready to get crazy, I'm there for you as well. Good biking and good hacking!

Bicycles are big. Most of us grew up with them and learned to ride as children. There are an estimated 1 billion bikes on the planet.

A good chunk of that billion seems to reside in my garage.

That's kind of the joke about bikes, right? You always seem to collect old and busted ones, which end up clogging your storage space until they get donated, sold, or thrown out *en masse*. This is especially true about kids' bikes, which are much cheaper and easier to replace than adult models, and consequently accumulate faster. It's less money to buy a new sweatshop-made kid's bike (like the one pictured in Figure 1-1) than it is to get that bike's wheel repaired in a bike shop. Between the cost of labor and parts, why not just buy new? On the other end of the spectrum, there are the hipster cruisers often selling for upwards of $1,000 apiece. These are not bikes you would hesitate to fix.

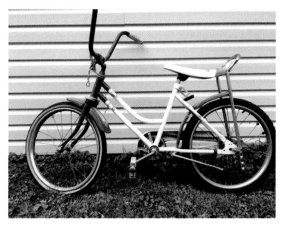

Figure 1-1 *This kiddie bike is crying out to be hacked!*

There is a beautiful middle ground between buying cheap junk not worth repairing, and buying expensive hardware you can barely afford. The solution is to make and modify your own bicycle. This book shows you how, ranging from welding up a frame to converting your regular bike into a cargo bike capable of hauling a couple bags of groceries. Along the way, you'll explore electronics, build a bike horn, add LED effects, and complete a bunch more projects to make your bike uniquely yours.

Bikes are everywhere. Find one and make it your own.

Origins

The bicycle was developed over time by many different inventors and mechanics across the world, with each person contributing a few new ideas to what became a very cool invention. The original two-wheeled, human-powered bike was the "Dandy Horse," introduced in Mannheim in 1817 and Paris in 1818. It resembled a bike without pedals, chains, or gears, and it was propelled, Fred Flintstone-like, by the rider's feet running along the ground. It took several false starts before bike makers settled on the now-classic configuration.

One of the most memorable was the iconic Penny Farthing bicycle shown in Figure 1-2, which flourished for barely a dozen years in the late 1870s and 1880s. While just a fad, the Penny Farthing became a symbol of the Victorian era, and its technology lives on: bike makers' attempts to find the perfect wheel ratios led to the adoption of the chain drive as the go-to method of propulsion, and those ratios still exist today.

The creation of the chain drive, and its adoption by bicycle manufacturers, had in effect created a recognized standard bicycle: two wheels of identical size, with a metal frame connecting the wheels, and a sprocket equipped with pedals positioned between them. The cyclist sits on a saddle attached to the frame, and his or her pedaling energy is transmitted to the rear wheel with the help of a chain drive.

About the same time that this standard settled into place, around the end of the 19th century, a full-fledged bike craze began sweeping the world.

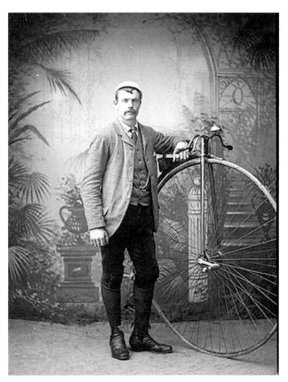

Figure 1-2 *The Penny Farthing was a popular configuration of bicycle in the late 1800s*

Anatomy of a Bicycle

Taking those configurations into consideration, a bicycle still boils down to a basic set of components: two wheels (usually), a frame to connect them, a place to sit, a braking system, and a set of pedals connected to an axle with a chain to drive the whole thing. Let's now review the various parts of the classic bike.

Brakes

The things that slow your bike down. Most adult bikes use cable brakes like the set shown in Figure 1-3. Another type is the coaster brake, the classic feature of kids' bikes. Well-heeled bike riders also dabble in disc brakes, which work by grabbing a disc mounted parallel to the wheel, rather than grabbing the wheel itself. Some cyclists remove the brakes altogether, preferring to rely on their biking skills to slow down in a hurry.

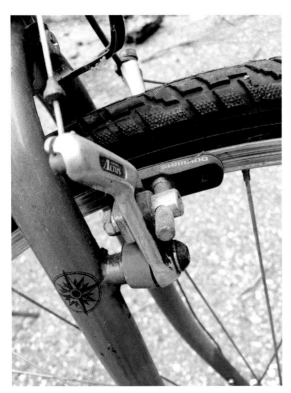

Figure 1-3 *Stop your bike on command with a set of brakes*

Brake Lever

You can control your brakes with these handle-bar-mounted levers. Like the model shown in Figure 1-4, brake levers are usually constructed to be gracefully curved, in order to be comfortable to grip for long periods of time.

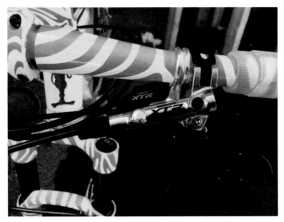

Figure 1-4 *Squeeze the lever to slow down the bike*

Cassette

When you hear about a bike having speeds, what this means is that it has multiple gears of different sizes. A big gear is slow, but has a lot of turning power to get you up hills. By contrast, a small gear is much faster, but doesn't have the torque to do the same hill. The cassette is the stack of gears on your bike, like the ones seen in Figure 1-5.

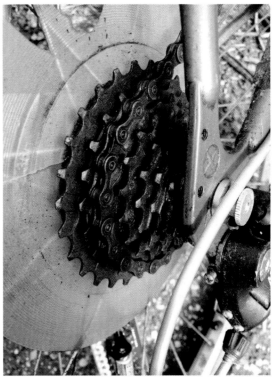

Figure 1-5 *The cassette is the stack of gears that the derailleur interacts with*

Chain

Made of interlocking metal links, the bike's chain (Figure 1-6) is a flexible way to transmit energy from the pedals to the wheels, and thereby move the bike. Because it's made up of links, you can make it whatever length you want. This will prove very convenient when you start hacking frames!

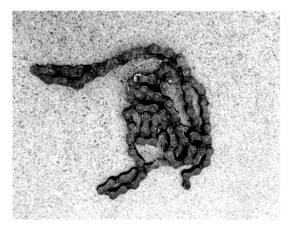

Figure 1-6 *A bike chain allows you to turn the rear wheel with the pedals*

Chainring

A chainring is the big gear that pedals are mounted to, as shown in Figure 1-7. It is this gear that moves the chain, because the cassette is mounted to it. The one shown here has been customized with a stenciled paint job.

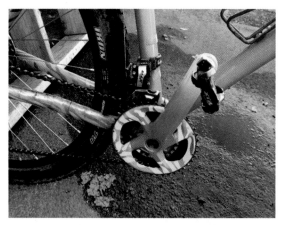

Figure 1-7 *Chainrings turn the chain as you pedal*

Derailleurs

These are the widgets that move the chain from one gear to the next, increasing and decreasing torque and speed (sort of like the transmission in a car). So-called "10-speeds" usually have front and back derailleurs, while bikes with fewer speeds might only have a single derailleur. And fixies do away with them altogether, forcing their riders to make do with a

single speed. You can see a derailleur in Figure 1-8.

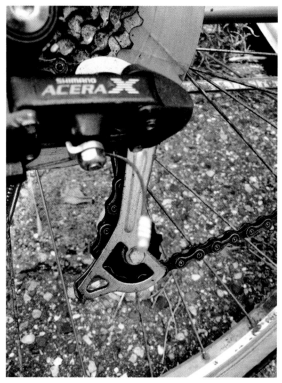

Figure 1-8 *Derailleurs control the chains, allowing you to switch speeds while moving*

Frame

The frame (Figure 1-9) is the chassis onto which all of the other parts of the bike are affixed. Typically it's made of welded steel tubing, giving it strength but relative lightness. However, many other materials are possible, ranging from "retro" all-wood frames to ultralight carbon-fiber models. In Chapter 7, we'll delve into frames big time, exploring the different parts of the frame and learning how to weld one of our own.

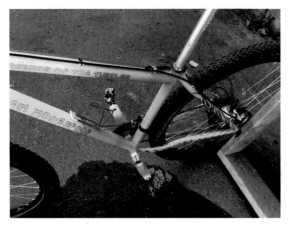

Figure 1-9 *Your bike frame keeps the bike's moving parts in order*

Gear Shifts

These controllers interact with the derailleurs to switch gears, enabling you to adjust the gear ratios to allow you to have more or less torque, depending on the riding conditions. Sometimes gear shifts look like little levers, like the ones shown in Figure 1-10, while other types are knobs on the handles.

Handlebars

It turns out that holding on to your bike is super important, and because of this, you'll find a wide variety of handlebar styles depending on what type of bike you're looking at, as well as the preferences of its owner. Mountain bikes, like the one pictured in Figure 1-11, use straight handlebars.

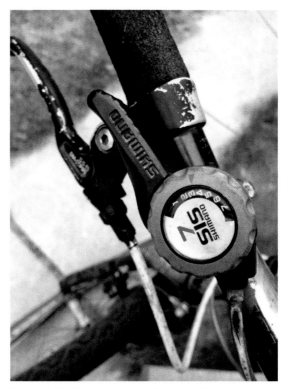

Figure 1-10 *Gear shifts control the derailleurs and allow you to move the chain from one gear to the next*

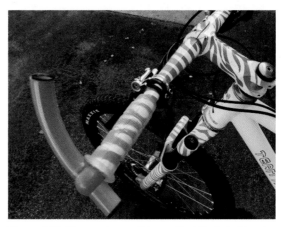

Figure 1-11 *You need something on the bike to hold on to —let's make it as comfortable as possible!*

Pedals

Every bike comes with pedals. Not surprisingly, there are a million different types of pedal and some are quite specialized. Racers favor racing cleats that prevent your shoes from slipping off the pedals, while others use radical friction, like the Odyssey pedals in Figure 1-12, to accomplish the same task.

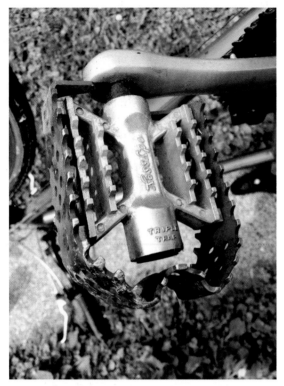

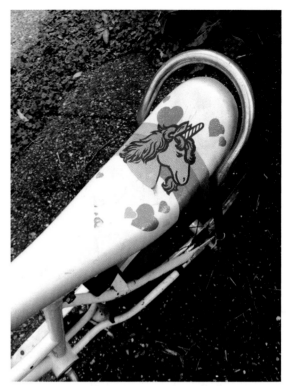

Figure 1-13 *A comfortable saddle, particularly one adorned with a unicorn, makes the bike experience more enjoyable*

Figure 1-12 *These cool pedals may kill your shins, but your feet won't slip off*

Saddle

Also known as the bike's seat, the saddle (Figure 1-13) is another part of the bike that is quickly switched out for a nicer upgrade or more customized configuration. Some seats are more padded, with gel packs making it more comfortable to sit for a long period of time. Racing saddles are made as light and aerodynamic as possible, at the price of not being as comfy.

Tires

Tires (Figure 1-14) are a pain to maintain—you have to pump them up, and sometimes they rupture no matter how carefully you avoid debris in the street. That said, a good set can make the bike-riding experience much smoother and more comfortable, not to mention safer. In Chapter 6, you'll have the opportunity to learn more about them.

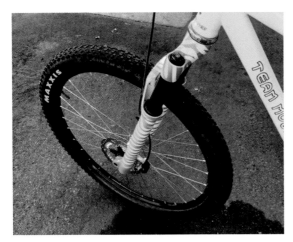

Figure 1-14 *Choose the right tires for your terrain*

Variants

Back in the late 1800s and early 1900s, in those first few heady decades of hacking, bicycle builders tried out countless variations of the two-wheel-balancing-vehicle combination, before eventually settling on the configuration we're accustomed to seeing. These days, bikes come in lots of different shapes and arrangements, taking advantage of the fact that we are all unique and have differing needs when it comes to a bike.

This book assumes you'll be working on a bike with the standard configuration: two wheels of equal size (often around 26" in diameter), a saddle on which you sit, handlebars to steer the front wheel, and pedals connected to a gearing system to make it move. Most of the options in the bike store will have the same style. Chances are every bike you have in your garage follows this design. Don't let that faze you! Check out these other types of bike that you're likely to encounter.

BMX

These bikes feature smaller-than-average wheels, often with plastic spokes. They are named for Bicycle Motorcross (with the "X" standing in for "cross") racing, where competitors jump their bikes and perform other stunts while racing around a dirt track. Because of this need for athleticism, BMX bikes also have a smaller frame size than standard bikes, looking like—or actually being—a kid's bike. Despite this, many adults ride BMXes out of nostalgia or simply for the fun of it.

Fixie

These are standard bikes with all the bells and whistles taken out—no derailleurs (gear shifting mechanisms), and just one speed. They are sometimes favored by expert riders who see no need for all those gadgets, needing only their instincts and experience to get them past obstacles.

Folding

These bikes are intended to be transported compactly, and therefore their frames fold down. That, plus the smaller wheel size, make them easier to store in an apartment closet, for instance.

Penny Farthing

As mentioned earlier, this classic design is marked by a huge front wheel and a smaller back wheel. It's not a very good design, which explains why it has gone out of popularity. However, historically minded DIYers and, dare I say it, hipsters have brought them back to a degree.

Recumbent

This bike has the cyclist sitting in a chair while working pedals at the front of the bike. This puts the rider very close to the ground, necessitating a pole and flag to ensure that passing motorists can see the vehicle and won't crush it.

Tall

On a tall bike, the frame is extended to absurd proportions, so the cyclist can't reach the ground with his or her feet. This necessitates holding on to trees and poles when the bike isn't in motion.

Tandem

A bicycle built for two! Usually the front person steers, while the back handlebars are fixed and just there for the back person to hold on to. Both cyclists pedal the bike.

Tricycle

Yes, there are grown-up–sized trikes. They offer an increased stability for riders who might not be so confident about balancing. In addition, they have more room for cargo.

Unicycle

A class mode of transportation for clowns and other circus performers, the unicycle is notoriously difficult to master, due to having to balance left and right while simultaneously keeping the bike from flipping forward or backward.

Just Hack It

Hacking is the opposite of that beautiful, gleaming $2,000 bike. Which is not to say its beauty isn't really worth two grand—but I'd never want to hack it. Consider instead that old beater, like the one shown in Figure 1-15. It's crying out for a new paint job, a cargo trailer, or possibly something even more exciting (maybe a way to generate electricity, a smartphone rig, or a sweet LED headlight?). With that junker, you get the freedom to play and hack without damaging something expensive.

Bike hacking is nothing more than modifying your bike to work better for you, fixing it when repairs are needed, and otherwise making it more your own. In a sense, it's taking total ownership of your bicycle—as well you should, considering your safety and your transportation needs depend on it. It also enables you to fix it more readily. Once you've stripped down and reassembled a bicycle, chances are nothing about its repair will stymie you.

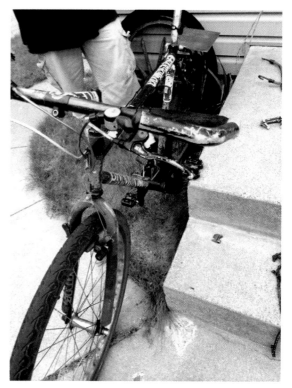

Figure 1-15 *This old beater has better days ahead of it*

More importantly, once you've fixed and modded a junker, you'll be liberated to do pretty much anything with your bike. It can be something as simple as installing new reflectors, or as complex as building an Arduino-powered lighting system.

Just hack it.

Summary

Chapter 1 got you going with a full-on immersion in bike 101. In Chapter 2, you'll hack right away with a number of simple customizations anyone can do.

Basic Bike Mods

2

Hacking, especially on an expensive or irreplaceable bike, can intimidate even an experienced tinkerer. This chapter is all about some super basic bike hacks pretty much anyone can do. Once you get your feet wet with these, you'll be primed to try something more challenging. Consider the SpokePOV, an electronic kit (seen in Figure 2-1) you can solder together and add to your bike. It is a reasonably challenging build that is certain to embolden you to do more cool stuff to your bike. In this chapter, we'll check out a number of similarly easy mods.

Commercial Add-Ons

The easiest form of bike modification is simply to buy a kit, of course. Examples include lights, horns, more comfortable seats, replacement pedals, and so on. In this section, we'll review a sampling of products that can be purchased and added on to your bike. In later chapters, I'll show you how to build DIY versions of a lot of these products.

Bottle Holder

The classic bike mod: adding a beverage holder. It's quick, it's easy, and it's a project that kids can do pretty well. A lot of bikes come with a bottle holder already installed (like the one

shown in Figure 2-2) but that doesn't mean it works the way you like it. Swap in a different bottle clip, or better yet, design your own!

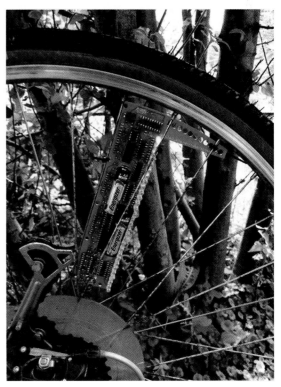

Figure 2-1 *The SpokePOV adds cool LED effects to your bike*

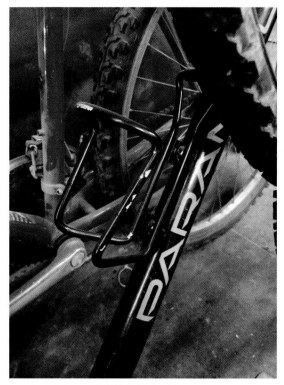

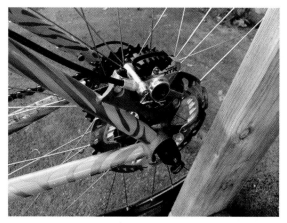

Figure 2-3 *Though pricey, disc brakes offer an improvement in braking ability*

Figure 2-2 *A beverage holder is the classic bike mod*

Brakes

Swapping in higher-end brakes, like the sweet disc brakes pictured in Figure 2-3, is a great way to improve your bike beyond its default equipment. You don't have to go quite so high-end; simply buying a slightly better-than-stock pair of standard brakes will benefit you by making your ride a little safer.

Cargo

Since the beginning of bicycling, folks have thought up ways to haul stuff using their bikes. Even if it's as simple as the child's basket shown in Figure 2-4, it's always useful to have a place on your bike to put stuff. In Chapter 11, you'll have an opportunity to explore a couple of different projects that help you to lug stuff around.

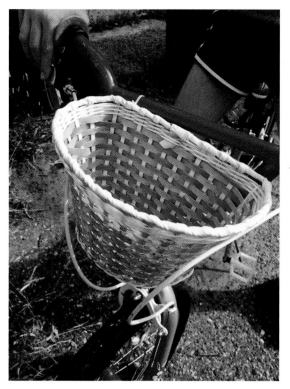

Figure 2-4 *Don't underestimate the importance of being able to carry stuff with your bike*

Child Seat

The classic add-on, prized by moms and dads as a way of getting their kids around in the summer. Child seats (Figure 2-5) often mount like a rack, with supports bolted to the rear axle.

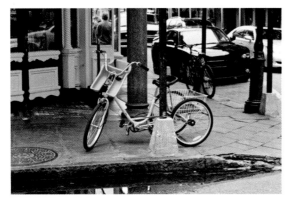

Figure 2-5 *A child seat lets you safely carry a small passenger*

Fenders

Fenders (Figure 2-6) are mostly there to keep mud from splashing up and making a dirty stripe up your back. If you ride your bike in inclement weather, you may want to get a fender. If you don't ride in the rain, you probably won't need one.

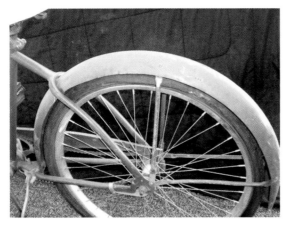

Figure 2-6 *Fenders keep rain and mud off your back (Photo credit: Alexis O'Toole, Creative Commons)*

Handlebars

You might not ordinarily identify a frame element like handlebars as something that is easily modifiable, but they are. For instance, you could trade your straight "mountain"-style han-

dlebars for ones that are more curved. Additionally, grips like the ones in Figure 2-7 can be added on to the ends of handlebars, giving you two ways to control your bike.

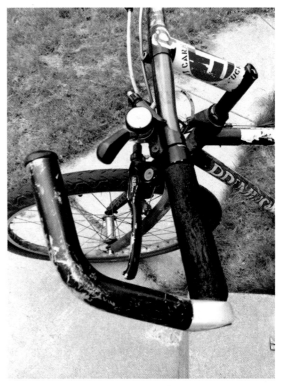

Figure 2-7 *What are the right handlebars for you?*

Lights

Headlights (like the light pictured in Figure 2-8) are considered a necessity for night riding, mostly so motorists can see you. In fact, taillights are arguably more important, as drivers approaching you from behind will see them before they see that you have a headlight.

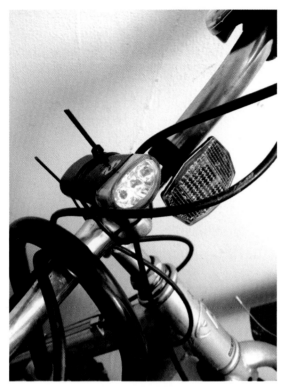

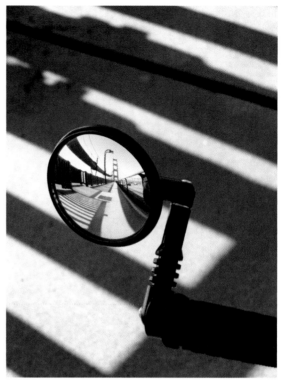

Figure 2-8 *Headlights show the way, and alert nearby motorists that you're there*

Figure 2-9 *Who's coming up behind you? (Photo credit: Dawn Endico, Creative Commons)*

Mirrors

Add-on mirrors, as seen in Figure 2-9, help cyclists keep an eye on the road behind them without turning their head. You'll often see mirrors bolted on to the ends of the handlebars, but there are also helmet-mounted options.

Noisemaker

The classic means for alerting pedestrians, a bell or horn, such as the one shown in Figure 2-10, can be easily added to your bike (the only tool you'll need is a screwdriver). But this category is not limited to warning-related bells and horns. For instance, there is an old-school bike mod consisting of a baseball card clothespinned to the bike axle. When the wheel turns, the card flaps against the spokes, making a vague engine noise. In Chapter 10, I show how to solder up your own electronic buzzer.

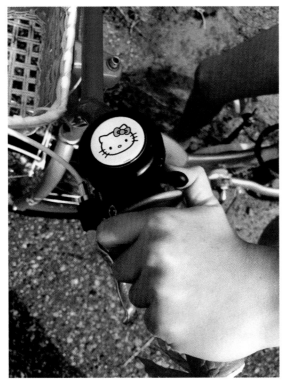

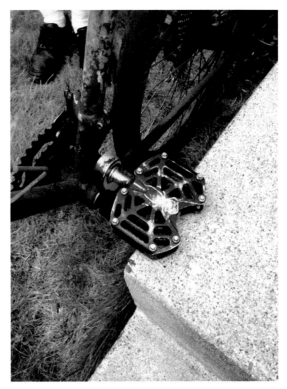

Figure 2-10 *Alert pedestrians with a horn or other noisemaker*

Figure 2-11 *These sweet pedals look great when your feet aren't covering them up*

Pedals

Customizing pedals is a great way to add utility, because there are many usage-related reasons why you'd want to switch them. As I mentioned, racers like to get special cleats that keep their feet from falling from the pedal during a competition. However, there are cosmetic pedals, like the sweet set shown in Figure 2-11, that merely add style to what would otherwise be a fairly boring part of your bike.

Pegs

Pegs (seen in Figure 2-12) are extensions screwed on to the axles of a bike. These allow the rider to do stunts and also make it easier for a passenger to ride along. You can find these dirt cheap, or you can get much nicer, artisanal pegs that cost more. This is another easy mod because you're just screwing on the peg as if it were a nut.

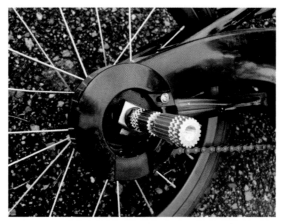

Figure 2-12 *Pegs give you a place to put your feet*

Reflectors

These headlight-reflecting panels are added to increase the bike's visibility at night. Most bikes come with reflectors already, but you can replace a missing or damaged one, or upgrade to a new and cooler set, like the one shown in Figure 2-13.

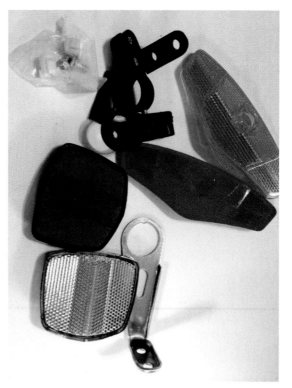

Figure 2-13 *Reflectors make your bike more visible at night*

Repair Kit

If you rely on your bike for transportation, not just for touring the neighborhood, you'll want a compact toolkit to carry with you, like the one shown in Figure 2-14. Even if it's just a patch kit and an Allen wrench, you may be very glad you packed one. Chapter 4 includes the inventory for an on-the-go bike repair kit.

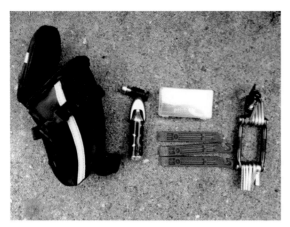

Figure 2-14 *This repair kit helps you solve minor—and sometimes major—problems on the road*

Saddle

Of course it's a cinch to buy a new saddle. They come in a vast array of shapes and padding levels. Some people go to absurd lengths to keep a specific type of seat that they like. The saddle in Figure 2-15 is a reproduction of a classic saddle, and its owner bought a couple dozen of them so he'd never have to use another type.

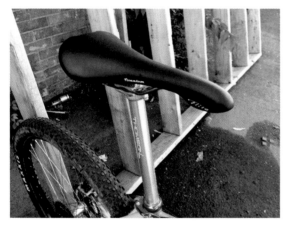

Figure 2-15 *A custom saddle boosts comfort and your bike's attractiveness*

Smartphone Mount

With the advent of the smartphone, there are seemingly limitless possibilities for using one in conjunction with your bike; of course, you'll want to pull over to the side of the road to respond to your friend's text message, though

there are hands-free navigation apps that allow you to stay on course as you ride. You can also use your smartphone to record your extreme mountain biking or other stunts. Commercial phone mounts, like the Hitcase mount seen in Figure 2-16, are readily available, but you can always build your own. Later in this chapter, I'll show you how to 3D-print a smartphone mount you can add to your bike.

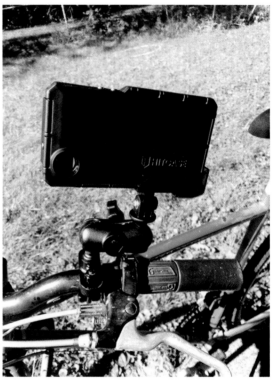

Figure 2-16 *This smartphone case positions your phone where it will be the most useful*

Stickers and Streamers

Stickers, such as the one shown in Figure 2-17, are an easy way to add personality to your bike. One of many sources for nerdy stickers is Adafruit (*http://www.adafruit.com/products/697*), which has "skill badge" stickers showing off your prowess with 3D printers, soldering irons, and other tools. Also in this category are streamers for your handlebars (whatever floats your boat!) and other strictly cosmetic additions.

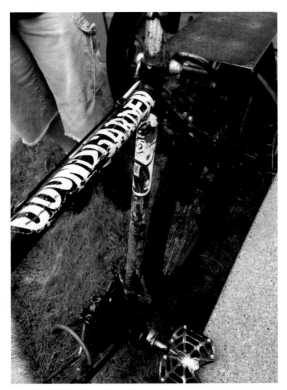

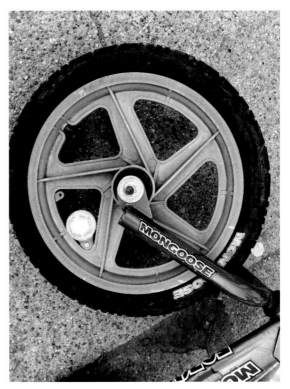

Figure 2-17 *Add stickers to your bike to add a little individual flair*

Figure 2-18 *Wheels give the cyclist the ability to navigate different terrains.*

Wheels

You can change your wheels almost as readily as anything else on your bike. Power users are accustomed to swapping out wheels based on the weather: for instance, installing street slicks (low-friction wheels) when the weather is good. Another variation is the classic BMX-style "magg" wheel, shown in Figure 2-18, which has five or six heavy plastic spokes rather than the usual metal ones. And some racers use solid, carbon-fiber disks with no spokes at all for wheels!

Project #1: Adding EL Wire

As you can see, you already have a number of simple, low-cost options for hacking your bicycle. In the following sections, however, we'll add some more complicated projects. I would classify these projects as marginally more difficult and expensive than screwing on a new headlight, though they're still very basic compared to some of the challenges you'll encounter later on in the book.

For our first project, you will add a fun light-up effect to a bike. Electro-luminescent (EL) wire is just that: wire that lights up when energized by an alternating current (AC), without heating up like most light sources. To make it portable, you'll need a gadget called an inverter (pictured in Figure 2-19) that converts the direct current (DC) you get from a battery into AC. They're tiny and inexpensive, making this project quite cheap. On the downside, the inverter emits a noticeable and not terribly pleasant hum.

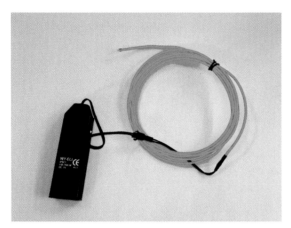

Figure 2-19 *EL wire makes a great visual effect for not a lot of money*

Parts List

This is a simple project and you'll only need a few parts:

- EL inverter: There are many to choose from, but I went with one from Spark-Fun, P/N 11222.

- EL wire: I chose blue EL wire from SparkFun, P/N 10195, but you should be able to find your favorite color of wire—Adafruit and SparkFun both have a variety of colors to choose from.

- Zip ties: Any that are long enough to fit around the tube; at least 5 inches. You can always cut off the end of a longer one!

Procedure

To add EL wire to your bike, follow along with these steps:

1. Zip-tie the inverter to a handy location on your bike, maybe the handlebars, as shown in Figure 2-20.

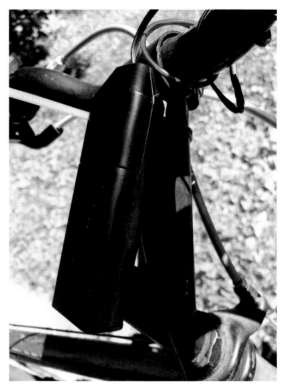

Figure 2-20 *Zip-tie the inverter*

2. Arrange the rest of the wire in an attractive way, zip-tying it as needed to various frame elements (Figure 2-21). You have 10 feet to work with, so have fun and be creative! Note that it does behave like wire, so once it gets bent it may not look as nice. No big deal! It will still light up.

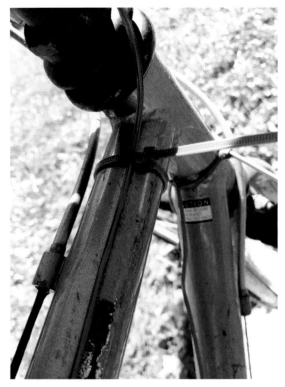

Figure 2-21 *Arrange the wire*

3. When you're done, turn on the inverter (preferably in the dark!), and check out your now glowing bike. If all goes well it should look like Figure 2-22.

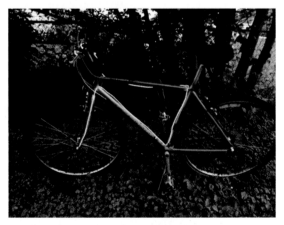

Figure 2-22 *Your bike glows in the dark!*

Project #2: Installing a SpokePOV Kit

Another way to add light to your bike is by using the SpokePOV, pictured in Figure 2-23. The name refers to "persistence of vision," a phenomenon where our minds "fill in the blanks" of images that exist only as the flashes of a LED light. Let's add a SpokePOV to your bike!

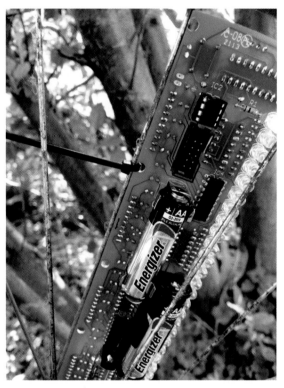

Figure 2-23 *The SpokePOV creates glowing images in your bike spokes*

Adafruit Industries created and sells the SpokePOV kit. It costs about $38 for red or yellow LEDs, or $45 with blue LEDs. Each kit features 60 LEDs, making it a fairly robust soldering job. If you don't know already, you can learn how to solder in Chapter 8.

Once assembled, the circuit board is attached to a wheel, so that when the wheel turns quickly, an image can be seen in the flashing lights of the spokes. If you install all three colors of SpokePOV on your wheel, you can create some crazy and colorful images!

Triggering the effect is a magnet you've strategically placed on the frame of the bike, close to where the SpokePOV turns. The magnet triggers the Hall effect sensor on the circuit board, which controls the speed at which the LEDs blink.

One cool aspect of the kit is that it can be cut down to fit a smaller wheel. If you have a BMX or kid's bike, you can saw off part of the PCB with a hacksaw or a similar cutting tool. One of the battery packs gets cut off along with some LED drivers and LEDs, but it works the same!

The SpokePOV comes with default images loaded onto it (including the biohazard symbol), as we'll soon see, but you can also program your own. This is actually rather tricky and requires a programming dongle like the USBtinyISP kit (Adafruit, P/N 46), or the equivalent components breadboarded up. The SpokePOV site (*http://www.ladyada.net/make/spokepov/*) has all the instructions you need to program it, as well as steps guiding you through assembly and installation.

Parts List

You'll need the following parts to install the SpokePOV:

- SpokePOV Kit (P/N 5): Note that putting this together requires soldering; if you don't know how to solder, check out the how-to in Chapter 4.

- Magnet: I suggest going with Adafruit's recommended magnet, P/N 9; don't assume some old magnet you have lying around will be strong enough to trip the Hall effect sensor—I did, and it didn't work.

- Zip ties: Get ties long enough to reach around the circumference of the tube —7" ties do the trick.

Procedure

Skipping over the soldering parts, which Adafruit describes on its site, let's instead begin with a finished SpokePOV:

1. Put the POV on either your front or back wheel—or both, if you have two kits. The point on the PCB should be pointing back, and the curved part should be against the rim.

2. Secure the circuit board to the spokes with zip ties, as shown in Figure 2-24. Don't worry, there are plenty of mounting holes on the board.

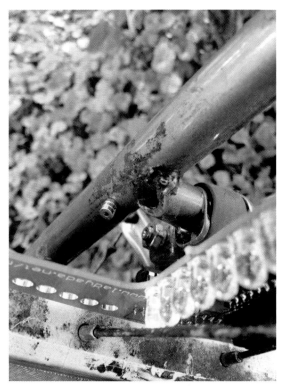

Figure 2-24 *Zip-tie the SpokePOV to the spokes*

3. Place the magnet (Figure 2-25) on one of the frame parts that will bring it close to the Hall effect sensor on the circuit board. This is easy to test— when the batteries are in the Spoke-POV and the Hall effect sensor detects a magnet, the LEDs will go crazy, flash-

ing as they attempt to create an image. When you're able to trigger the LEDs just by turning the wheel, you'll know you've got it right.

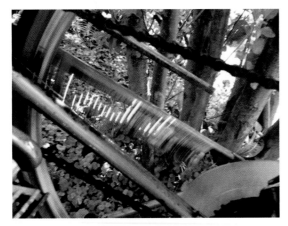

Figure 2-25 *A magnet triggers the Hall effect sensor and activates the LED animation*

4. Like the EL wire, the SpokePOV looks best in the dusk or at night. Test it out! Figure 2-26 shows how it should look.

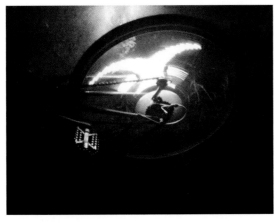

Figure 2-26 *You've never been so happy to see a biohazard symbol!*

Project #3: DIY Smartphone Rig

This phone clip is one of a gazillion smartphone rigs that you can make on a 3D printer. It was designed by Sven Van Dam of Umake (*http://*

www.umake.nl) and you can download it from the project page (*http://www.thingiverse.com/thing:214436*), which is hosted by 3D-printing resource Thingiverse.

Creating this rig assumes you have access to a 3D printer, which might not always be the case. On the other hand, you might be surprised to hear that you may be able to access one very close to you. Libraries, Maker spaces, community colleges, and other organizations offer classes in 3D printing, and allow visitors to use the equipment. You can even order a print of a 3D object through online printing services like Shapeways (*http://www.shapeways.com*). If you are new to 3D printing, *Make:* has an excellent resource for learning the ropes. It's called *Getting Started with Makerbot* and it can guide you through all the steps of 3D printing from the design process through to the output.

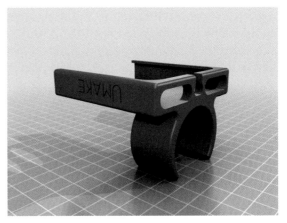

Figure 2-27 *This iPhone holder clips on to the bike's frame (Photo credit: Sven Van Dam/Umake)*

Procedure

Follow along with these steps to print your phone clip:

1. Download the clip from the Thingiverse project page (*http://www.thingiverse.com/thing:214436*), and print it out on your 3D printer.

2. Clip it on your bike.

3. Insert your iPhone 5 or 5S (Figure 2-28) to have a handy navigation display while on the road.

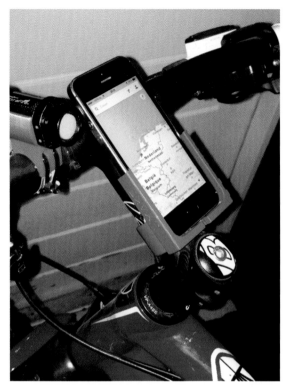

Figure 2-28 *The phone rig lets you navigate while riding (Photo credit: Sven Van Dam/Umake)*

If you want a holder for some other kind of phone, chances are someone has already designed one. Search on Thingiverse for your phone's model number and see what you come up with. If not, learn a 3D-design program like SketchUp (*http://www.sketchup.com*) and design it yourself!

Summary

In this chapter, we learned about some very basic modifications that mostly anyone with a screwdriver and a little money can do. In Chapter 3, I'm going to kickstart your hacking mood by showing you some of the cool rides that bike hackers have created.

Gallery of Cool Bikes

3

Now that you've had a chance to get in the bike-hacking mindset, here's some inspiration: a dozen interesting bikes that have been (or are screaming to be!) hacked and modded.

Unicycle Conversion

Peter Wagner converted a typical unicycle (Figure 3-1) into a mini bike by bolting on a set of handlebars and a child-size front wheel. Best of all, if you loosen some bolts, the front pops off easily, restoring it to its one-wheeled glory.

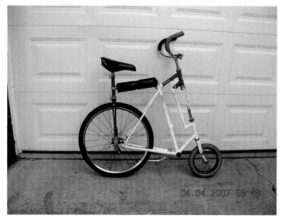

Figure 3-1 *A unicycle conversion made from combining two bikes (Photo credit: Peter Wm. Wagner, aka Whymcycles)*

This project exemplifies the possibilities of hacking a bike's frame, mixing and matching parts to create new and crazy variants. In Chapter 7, I offer tips on doing just that, as well as walking you through the steps to weld up your own.

Chopper Bike

The Puch Chopper shown in Figure 3-2 is begging to get hacked! Sometimes quirky old bikes like this one make the best fodder for modification.

I'd love to see the seat itself get reupholstered, maybe vinyl with some swank '70s pattern. The wheels could use a refresh as well, looking kind of sad…maybe some knobby offroaders would work. However, I wouldn't repaint the lovely frame for the world.

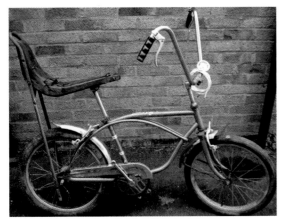

Figure 3-2 *Who wants to mod this classic bike? (Photo credit: Warren Cox)*

Stretch Cruiser Bike

Gerry Lauzon's cruiser bike (Figure 3-3) was created by welding together two different frames, making it especially long. This "Frankensteining" of multiple bikes is a common approach in the bike-hacking world.

Think about it—metal pipes are more than strong enough to support your weight, so as long as the frame still functions correctly from a mechanical aspect, you can get away with some unusual configurations.

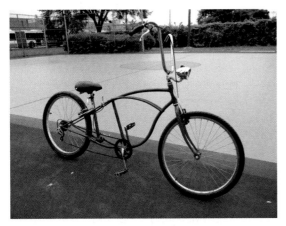

Figure 3-3 *You can make a really long bike out of two normal bikes! (Photo credit: Gerry Lauzon, Creative Commons)*

Restored Cruiser

Nathan Proudlove welded a decorative plate of steel on to an old bike (Figure 3-4) and replaced the wheels, saddle, and handlebars. Then he gave the bike a beautiful paint job. When that was all done, he made it into a fixie.

Some Makers absolutely love finishing their creations with fine details like stained hardwood, brass hardware, and tasteful paint. This is the bike equivalent, with hand-painted trim matching the rims on the tires.

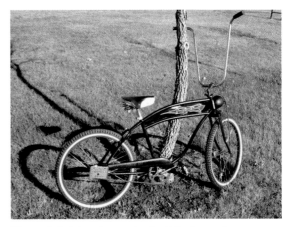

Figure 3-4 *Sometimes a hacked bike is nearly indistinguishable from a new one! (Photo credit: Nathan Proudlove)*

High Rider

Garret Farmer and Gabriel Kaprielian built this "high rider" bike (Figure 3-5), so called because it resembles a normal bike in its configuration, only taller. It is part of a larger category of bikes with oversized frames, called tall bikes.

This is another example of Makers combining two frames to create a new one. The white portion is from one frame; it is a step-through frame often associated with women's bikes. The seat tube is welded to the blue frame, about where the head tube is located. However, a crankset has been added here and the place where you'd ordinarily expect it to be, the bottom bracket, is just a hole in the frame.

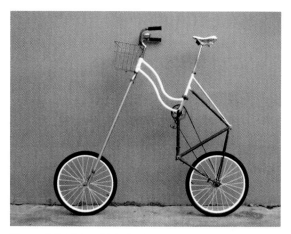

Figure 3-5 *This tall bike looks a lot like a normal bike, only taller! (Photo credit: Gabriel Kaprielian)*

Drift Trike

A subset of the DIY bikes scene involves building "drift trikes" (like the one pictured in Figure 3-6), which are grown-up–sized Big Wheel–style trikes, equipped with plastic tubes covering the treads of the rear tires, allowing some fun sliding stunts.

This is an example of a subset of Making where an entire subculture develops around one particular set of hacks. You can learn a lot from folks who have built a few of these trikes—but only if you can adapt that specialized knowledge to suit your project.

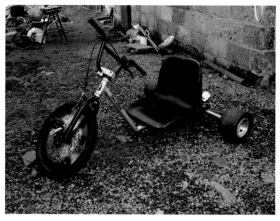

Figure 3-6 *This drift trike lets you do stunts (Photo credit: DrQuiMobile, public domain)*

Cargo Bike

The sweet ride pictured in Figure 3-7 was hacked together from bike parts. The creator hacked off the bottom bracket, seat tube, and stays from the frame of a bike. A horizontal tube was welded to the bottom bracket and a diagonal support tube connected to the top of the seat tube. The end of the horizontal tube is a bearing of some sort, allowing the rider to turn the front wheel assembly and thereby steer the bike.

The cargo platform was attached using thin strips of metal resembling leaf springs, and this probably lends the platform a bit of shock absorption. The cargo area itself is a plain box of welded sheet steel. The lack of any bungee attachment lugs—not to mention the coaster brakes—suggests to me that this thing doesn't go very fast. I'll create my own variant of the cargo-hauling bike trailer in Chapter 11.

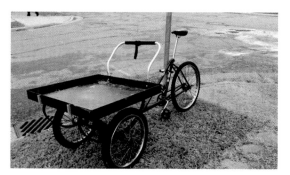

Figure 3-7 *Cargo bikes haul goods, ordinarily an iffy prospect in the bike world (Photo credit: Barbara Baichtal)*

Bouncer

Peter Wagner's bounce-powered roller (he calls them Whymcycles—pronounced "whimsicals") includes sports car tires and a robust welded frame. The rider jumps up and down on the horizontal bar in the middle (Figure 3-8) and this turns a mechanism inside the rear wheel that makes the bike go forward.

Peter's creations are often seen in parades (certain parades and festivals are a great place to find excellently hacked bikes, and to connect with people who are exploring the boundaries of what bikes are all about).

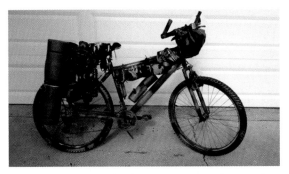

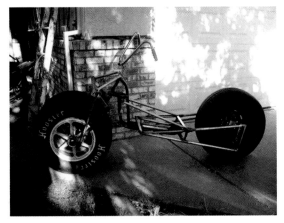

Figure 3-8 *Peter Wagner's Whymcycle moves when the rider bounces on it (Photo credit: Peter Wm. Wagner, aka Whymcycles)*

Bug-Out Bike

What will you ride when civilization falls? Ty Gladden modified his bike to be his post-apocalyptic transportation (*http://bit.ly/1NOMcjo*). In addition to the cool camo paint job (seen in Figure 3-9), the bike features panniers, a tent, and a mess kit, as well as a metal mailbox holding a pair of binoculars. It's just a clever picnic basket on wheels for Ty and his girlfriend.

In Chapter 12, I try something similar, only I'm creating a bike that combines a speaker, a light show, and a cooler for drinks!

Figure 3-9 *The Bug-Out Bike is more properly named the "Picnic Bike" (Photo credit: Ty Gladden)*

Parade Bike

This bike has a built-in sound system complete with amp and speakers, as well as a disco ball (barely visible in Figure 3-10). This bike falls into the category of parade bikes—improbably huge and ornate bicycles hauled out for the local parade.

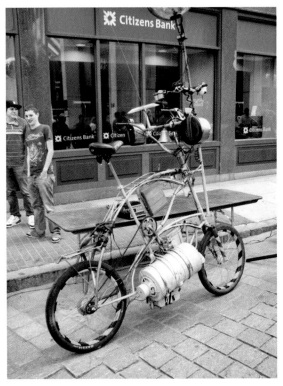

Figure 3-10 *This mobile sound system also works as a bike (Photo credit: Chris Connors)*

In this book, I dabble with a couple of audio-related projects, including a handlebar-mounted synthesizer horn (for more on this, flip to Chapter 10) as well as a light organ that responds to music being played nearby (we'll build this in Chapter 12).

Bike Plus Tape

Bike hacks don't have to involve welding or electronics. The bike in Figure 3-11 was made positively floral with the addition of some attractively arranged tape. Even better, it's temporary, so you can try out another idea any time you want.

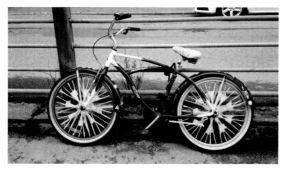

Figure 3-11 *A roll of tape can do wonders to dress up a bike (Photo credit: Hugo van Kemenade)*

This brings up a hesitation some Makers experience when thinking about hacking on their bike. What if they make the bike unrideable or mar its appearance? A temporary bike project like this one is the answer.

Kinetic Sculpture Racer

The vehicle shown in Figure 3-12 is made to travel on both water and ground, using large wheels studded with paddles, while employing large plastic wheels (not shown) for flotation. Meanwhile, the front wheel serves as a rudder.

The bicycle is the perfect human-powered vehicle, and you can see how Makers use it as a starting point for other hacks. Imagine looking at a bike and trying to figure out how to make a boat out of it, while still retaining its ability to roll like a bike. Challenges like that inspire Makers to design and construct some pretty cool creations.

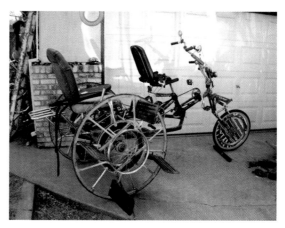

Figure 3-12 *This three-wheeled vehicle converts to a paddleboat (Photo credit: Peter Wm. Wagner, aka Whymcycles)*

Summary

How can you not be inspired by all of these cool bikes? In later chapters, you'll learn how to make a bunch of cool projects, but in the meantime, you still have more skills to master. In Chapter 4, you'll learn about a variety of tools used by bike-hackers, including specialized wrenches used for just one part, as well as commonplace tools you'll need all the time.

Bike Hacker's Workbench

4

Before you start in on the challenging projects, let's review some of the tools and techniques you'll need. You'll have the opportunity to check out a couple of different toolkits, one for home and one for on the road. This will give you a solid base of tools that will allow you to safely disassemble anything on a bike.

The Essential Bike Mechanic's Toolkit

Nearly everything you need to work on a bike's mechanical parts fits into a small duffel bag. The following sections describe what you should grab.

Bike Stand

Bikes, when not in motion, are inherently unstable, and trying to repair a bike while it's on its kickstand or (my personal favorite) upside down on its handlebars is asking for your bike to fall over. A bike stand, shown in Figure 4-1, is a heavy tripod with a strong gripper that keeps the bike elevated and steady while you work.

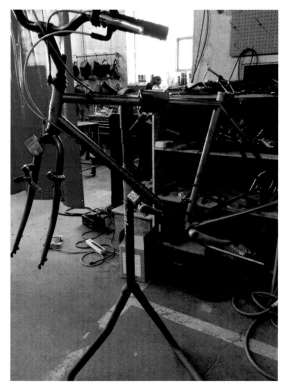

Figure 4-1 *The bike stand holds your bike so you don't have to*

Bottom Bracket Tool

The bottom bracket tool (Figure 4-2) is one of several specialized wrenches you'll need. This one removes the bottom bracket, the assembly

29

that connects the chainring and pedals to the frame.

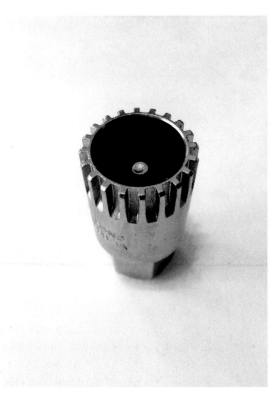

Figure 4-2 *You'll need the right tool to remove the bottom bracket*

Cable Cutter

A cable cutter (Figure 4-3) makes it easier to trim cables to the right size. Some also have a crimper to secure the nut to the end of the cable, to help inhibit frays.

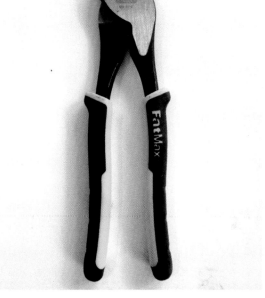

Figure 4-3 *A cable cutter helps cut neatly through cables and housings*

Cable Puller

Cable pullers (Figure 4-4) are multifunction tools for adjusting cables, allowing you to adjust your brakes exactly how tight you want them. They also work for securing zip ties, pulling them nice and snug.

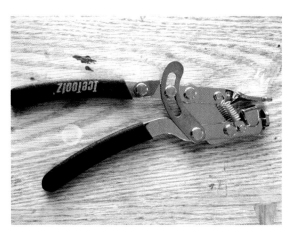

Figure 4-4 *The cable puller keeps the cable taut while you secure it*

Chain Breaker

The chain breaker (Figure 4-5) forces the rivet out of a bicycle chain, allowing you to replace, repair, or resize the chain.

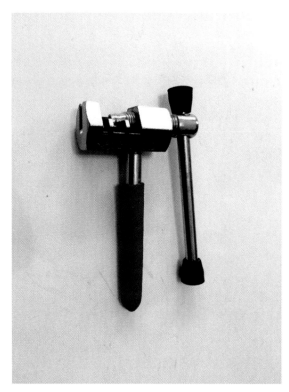

Figure 4-5 *The chain breaker is a necessity for working with chain links*

Chainring Nut Wrench

This wrench (seen in Figure 4-6) opens the specialized nuts that secure the chainring.

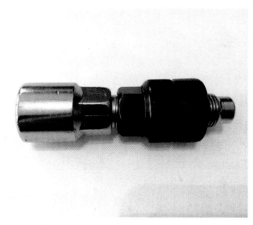

Figure 4-6 *The chainring nut wrench is a must for working with the bike's crankset.*

Chain Wear Indicator

It's hard to tell how worn your chain is getting without being able to compare it to something. The wear indicator (Figure 4-7) allows you to measure the chain's gauge to make sure it's still fit for use.

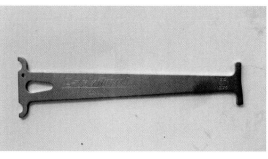

Figure 4-7 *The chain wear indicator helps you determine whether to replace your chain*

Chain Whip

A chain whip (Figure 4-8) is also known as a freewheel turner. It combines three tools into one: it has a pedal wrench on one end, and two chains on the other. One chain is fixed, while the other one is loose, giving you two ways to control your freewheel-enabled wheel while you work on it.

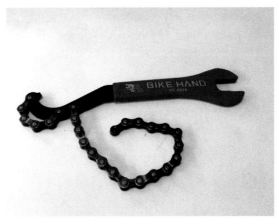

Figure 4-8 *A chain whip lets you keep a freewheel-equipped wheel from moving*

CO2 Inflator

If you have to inflate a tire on the road, there are two choices: hand pumps or a CO2 canister like the one in Figure 4-9. The inflator sits in your repair kit, and when you need to inflate a tire, just grab it! You can get multiple uses out of one canister, depending on how flat your tire is—it has enough CO2 to inflate one fully deflated tire.

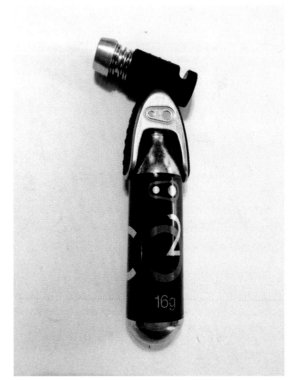

Figure 4-9 *This small capsule inflates your bike tire*

Cone Wrenches

Cone wrenches (Figure 4-10) look like normal key wrenches except much thinner. They're used to work on the wheel bearings, adjusting the part of the hub called the cone.

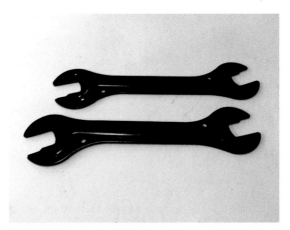

Figure 4-10 *Cone wrenches are used to adjust a bike wheel's hub*

Crank Puller

The crank puller (Figure 4-11) is a small wrench for removing the cranks, the arms that connect the pedals to the chainring.

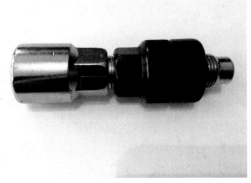

Figure 4-11 *Add or remove the cranks with this wrench*

Freewheel Remover

Like a lot of bike parts, you need a special wrench (Figure 4-12) to loosen the freewheel, a mechanism in the hub of the rear wheel.

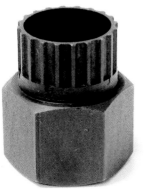

Figure 4-12 *Loosen or tighten the bike's freewheel with this wrench*

Grease

You want to use high-quality bicycle grease (Figure 4-13) to lubricate your axles.

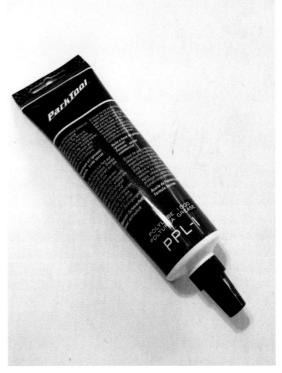

Figure 4-13 *Grease the wheel with a high-quality lubricant*

Hex Wrench

As mentioned, hex wrenches (often called Allen wrenches, shown in Figure 4-14) are commonly used in the biking world. A nice assortment—more than just what the multitool offers—will come in handy.

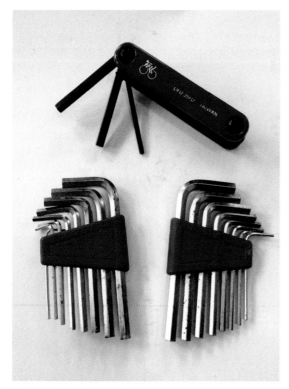

Figure 4-14 *Hex wrenches are an absolute necessity*

Key Wrench

The key wrench—the one in Figure 4-15 is 8mm—is an asset, and you won't regret keeping it in your toolbox. The specific size depends on the size of bolts your bike uses. You might just want to get a set!

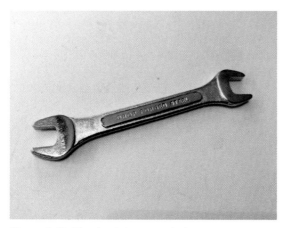

Figure 4-15 *The classic key wrench always comes in handy*

Lockring Remover

Yet another specialty wrench, this one (pictured in Figure 4-16) loosens the part that secures the cassette of gears.

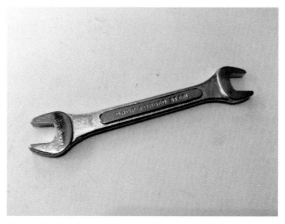

Figure 4-16 *The locking remover is another tool you'll only use for one bicycle part*

Multitool

Multitools in the bike world look a lot different than other multitools—no scissors or magnifying glass on this bad boy! Typically multitools have a bunch of hex bits in addition to a few other tools—the Crank Brothers multitool pictured in Figure 4-17 also has a chain breaker and pedal wrench built in.

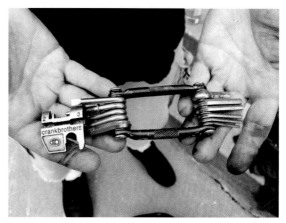

Figure 4-17 *Bicycle multitools: more than just a lot of hex wrenches*

Pedal Wrench

A wrench for loosening your pedals, shown in Figure 4-18. You'll often see pedal wrenches built into some other tool.

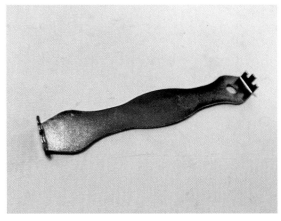

Figure 4-18 *Secure your pedals using a pedal wrench*

Pressure Gauge

Bike fanatics swear by keeping their tires properly inflated. Be sure to check your wheel's rating (often written near the valve) before you inflate, using a pressure gauge like the one in Figure 4-19.

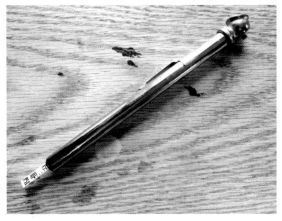

Figure 4-19 *Ensure proper wheel inflation with a pressure gauge*

Rasp and Patches

Unless you want to spring for a whole new inner tube, repairs often consist of gluing a piece of rubber—a patch—on your tube. A typical

kit, such as the one shown in Figure 4-20, includes a rasp for conditioning the area around the puncture, several patches, as well as a tube of glue.

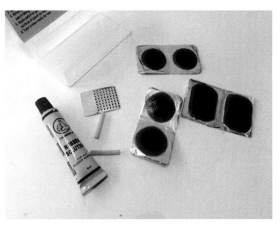

Figure 4-20 *Fixing flats requires a rasp and patches*

Screwdrivers

Though hex wrenches are commonplace in the bike world, you'll still need screwdrivers, both flat and Phillips. The screwdriver in Figure 4-21 is double ended so you can drive both types with one tool.

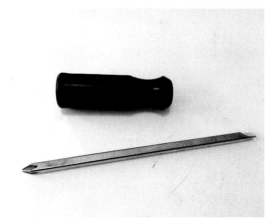

Figure 4-21 *Screwdrivers are still needed despite the preponderance of hex bolts*

Socket Set

Wrenches are all well and good, but sometimes you need a high-quality socket set. The set pictured in Figure 4-22 is great for removing stubborn hex bolts.

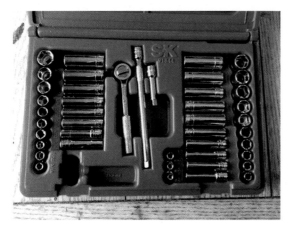

Figure 4-22 *A small socket set will often come in handy*

Spoke Wrench

The spoke wrench loosens or tightens the spoke's nipple, the hardware that secures the spoke to the rim. The wrench pictured in Figure 4-22 has slots to accommodate various spoke gauges.

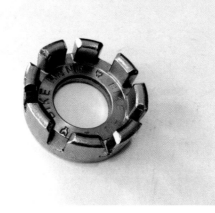

Figure 4-23 *A spoke wrench has grooves for various gauges of spoke*

Tire Levers

Tire levers, like the ones in Figure 4-24, help pry the tire away from the rim.

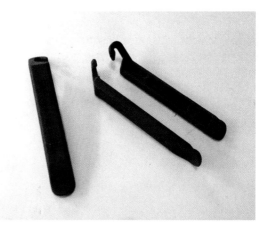

Figure 4-24 *Tire levers are a necessity for working on a bike tube*

Assembling the Ultimate On-the-Go Bike Repair Kit

Sometimes you don't want even a medium-sized toolkit—if you're on the road, you'll want your kit to be as light and slender as possible, something that will cover the likeliest emergencies. The good news is that you don't have to bring a bunch of stuff with you to tackle the two most likely repair tasks: fixing tires and tightening random bolts. The following toolkit (pictured in Figure 4-25) will help you accomplish both of these tasks without weighing you down:

- Container
- Multitool
- Tire levers
- Tire repair kit
- Air canister

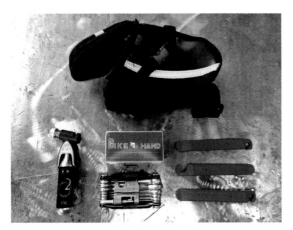

Figure 4-25 *Carry this toolkit with you when you're on the road*

Summary

In this chapter, we delved into the tools we need to work on bikes. It turns out that there are quite a lot of them! There are dozens of specialized parts that you might theoretically need, but also a relatively small set that are most commonly employed by bike hackers. Now that you've boned up on tools, let's put that knowledge to the test in Chapter 5 by trying out some rather intimidating mechanical tasks: stripping down your bike, painting it, and then rebuilding it as a fixed-gear bicycle.

Advanced Bike Mechanics

5

In this chapter, you'll get an opportunity to buff up on bike mechanics. First, you'll learn how to strip your bike down to its frame, removing everything from the saddle to the cables, kickstand, and derailleurs. The project following that involves repainting the frame, once you've removed all the accessories. Then we close out the chapter by showing how to reassemble your bike into a fixie, a bike without gear shifts and sometimes even without brakes. There's a lot to tackle! Let's get started.

Project #4: Stripping Down a Bike

The first project you'll tackle in this chapter is to strip down a bike. By that I mean removing all the hardware connected to the frame. This is not something you'll need to do all of the time, but especially if you're exploring customizing your bike, it's something you'll need to know *how* to do.

Parts List

- Tools: You'll need the toolkit discussed in Chapter 4.
- Degreaser: Any degreaser sold by a bike store will work.

- Cleaning supplies: All-purpose cleaning spray and paper towels.

Tips on Stripping Down Your Bike

The following are some suggestions to keep in mind when you begin your project:

Be gentle

Most of the time, everything on a bike is meant to be safely removed and replaced. However, if a bike has been left in the rain for a long time, or simply is very old, it's possible that parts that ordinarily could be easily removed are corroded or otherwise stuck in place. Maybe there's some grime or rust, or maybe the screws are stripped. If this is the case, you should remember that patience and gentleness are your allies.

Trying to force a stuck part may result in you damaging your bike by bending parts not meant to be bent. You might even permanently damage a part, which could sabotage your project by making your bike unrideable for a period of time. If a part isn't coming off, you can try squirting a ton of WD-40 or similar lubricant, coupled with some judicious taps of a hammer to knock it loose. If you start getting frustrated, step aside for a while!

Keep track of the hardware you remove

As you might have noticed from the list of wrenches in the previous chapter, seemingly every part on a bike has a different style of connector, and it's easy to mix them up. One tactic I've used is to take a photo of the hardware I removed so I know what the right connector looks like.

Be prepared to discover damage when you tear down your bike

Parts might be corroded or simply broken. While aluminum and stainless steel might be able to withstand a summer outdoors, many attachments—particularly third-party accessories—may be made of ordinary steel, which can't.

Assume you'll have to replace some of the more fragile parts on the bike

It's one thing to live with a busted cable, but putting it back on over a freshly cleaned bike is like putting on dirty clothes after a shower. It just feels wrong! If you're not happy putting a certain part back on the frame, be prepared to replace it. Fortunately, a lot of parts are fairly cheap.

If you're ready to begin, gather your tools together and get started!

Procedure

These are the steps you'll need to follow:

1. Begin by removing the saddle and other accessories that don't require tools to loosen. Basically, any accessory that has a quick release (like you can see in Figure 5-1) can be removed.

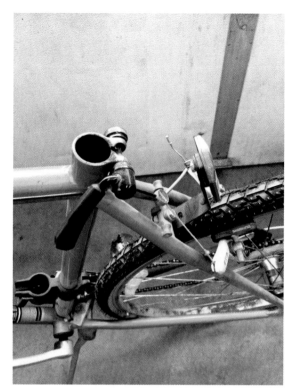

Figure 5-1 *Remove the saddle*

2. Next, bust out your tools and detach the remaining accessories: reflectors (shown in Figure 5-2), rack, basket, lights, and so on. Also, if the bike has fenders, remove them now. Remember that the hardware for these parts is likely to be stuck or rusted, particularly if it's an el-cheapo third-party product. Many of these have easily corroded hardware, making removal problematic.

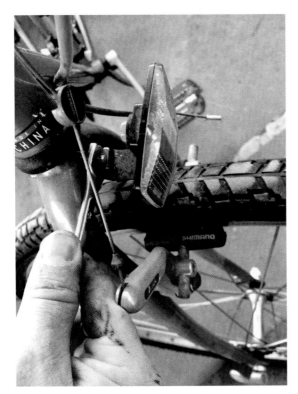

Figure 5-2 *Detach the reflectors and other easily removed accessories*

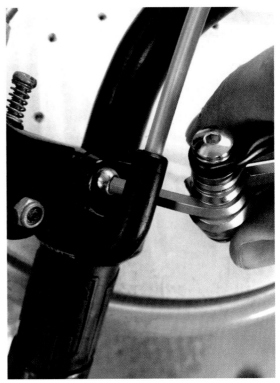

Figure 5-3 *Next, remove the gear shifts and brake levers*

3. Gear shifts and brake levers are next. Loosen the bolts attaching them to your handlebars (Figure 5-3) and let them dangle from their cables for now. If you intend to replace the cables, you can nip the cables close to the levers and simply remove them.

4. Remove the grips, including adhesive rubber, grip tape, and so on. Some grips bolt on (like the ones pictured in Figure 5-4) and therefore are easily removed. However, some are glued on and you'll have to scrape off some foam. Fun!

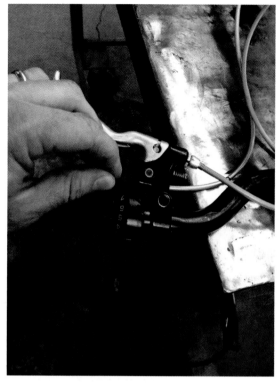

Figure 5-4 *Remove the grips*

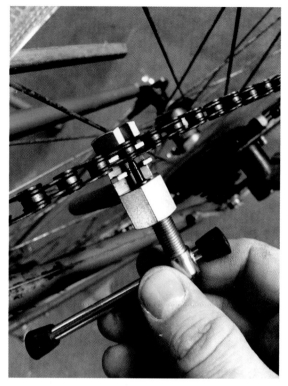

Figure 5-5 *Break the chain and remove it*

5. Remove the chain using a chain breaker. This involves tightening a threaded rod (Figure 5-5) so that it forces out the link's rivet. The chain is likely to be covered in grease, so you may want to protect yourself and your clothing from stains. This is a good opportunity to degrease the chain.

6. Remove the kickstand (Figure 5-6). You may have to flip the bike over to get at the bolt.

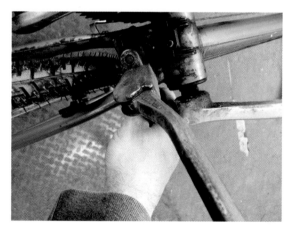

Figure 5-6 *Unbolt the kickstand*

7. Next, remove the front wheel, which often has a quick-release or other easily loosened hardware, seen in Figure 5-7.

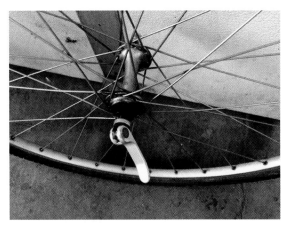

Figure 5-7 *The front wheel has a quick-release to help you remove it rapidly*

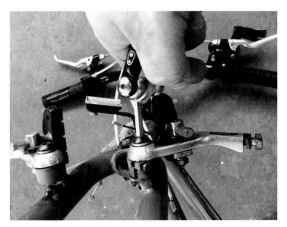

Figure 5-9 *Unbolt the brake mechanisms from the frame*

8. Remove the back wheel, seen in Figure 5-8. With the brakes disconnected and the chain removed, this is actually rather easy.

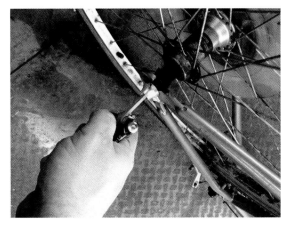

Figure 5-8 *Use a hex wrench to loosen the back wheel*

9. Finish removing the brakes, unscrewing the mechanisms from the frame, as seen in Figure 5-9.

10. Remove the brake and gear shift cables, using wire cutters as needed. I don't know about you, but I found tons of damage—frayed cables and cracked housings (Figure 5-10)—and you might want to assume you're going to have the same problem, so make sure you have some cables.

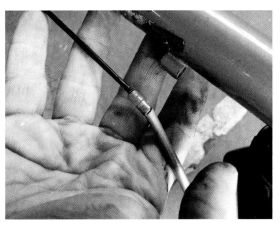

Figure 5-10 *I found lots of damage when I removed the cables*

11. Remove the front and back derailleurs, shown in Figure 5-11. Without the chains and cables installed, these should come off readily with a hex wrench.

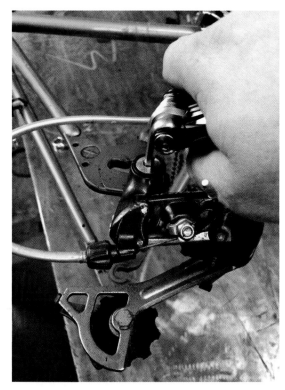

Figure 5-11 *Derailleurs are next*

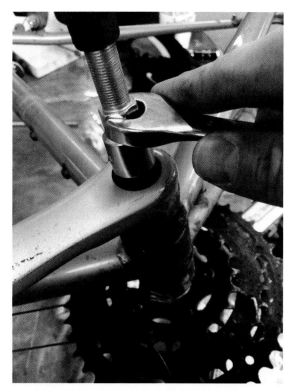

Figure 5-12 *Take off the pedals*

12. Next come the pedals. You can either remove the pedals from the cranks, or simply remove the cranks from the chainring and bottom bracket (Figure 5-12).

13. Unbolt the chainring from the bottom bracket (Figure 5-13). Some people don't bother removing the bottom bracket from the frame; unless it's in need of repair or replacement, you might want to just leave it in place. If you're painting the bike, simply tape over the hole—you wouldn't want paint in there no matter what.

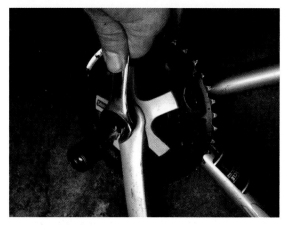

Figure 5-13 *Remove the chainring, leaving the bottom bracket in place*

14. Remove the handlebars and fork, shown in Figure 5-14.

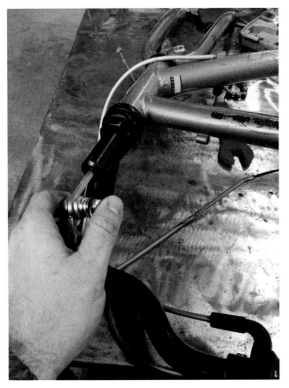

Figure 5-14 *Lastly, remove the handlebars and fork*

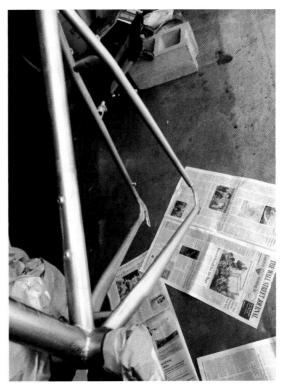

Figure 5-15 *It's time to paint your bike!*

15. You're done! Hopefully you kept track of your hardware and can put the bike back together again! On the other hand, you may want to take advantage of the bike's stripped-down state to paint it. If this is the case, read on.

Project #5: Painting a Bike

Once you've stripped down your bike, you have the option to paint it. It's not a bad idea. A can of spray paint is dirt cheap, and once you've removed all the parts from the frame, it's a cinch to throw on some paint and make it look brand new (Figure 5-15).

Parts List

- All-purpose cleaning spray
- Sandpaper
- Degreaser
- Painter's tape
- Spray paint

Procedure

Follow along with these steps to paint your bike:

1. Strip off the old stickers, adhesive, tape, and so on. Very often these will leave a gummy residue and this will need to come off as well. Then spray it down with regular, all-purpose cleaning spray (Figure 5-16) and scrub off the dirt. If your bike has seen a lot of use—particularly in grime or muck—chances are it

will need a nice scrub to get it clean. Additionally, you may need degreaser if there is a lot of built-up grease.

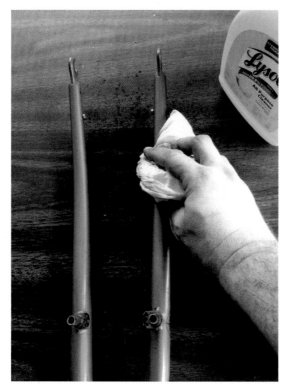

Figure 5-16 *Clean off all the grime*

2. Scuff up the surface of the existing paint job (Figure 5-17) with sandpaper. This will give the new coat of paint something to grip on to. Alternatively, you can attempt to remove the paint altogether.

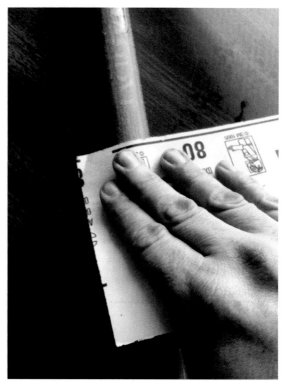

Figure 5-17 *Sand the surface of the existing paint job*

3. Tape off the bike, as shown in Figure 5-18. Once it's clean and dry, begin taping off the parts you don't want painted. These should include any mechanical parts you left on the bike (like the bottom bracket), any joints, connection holes, and threaded areas.

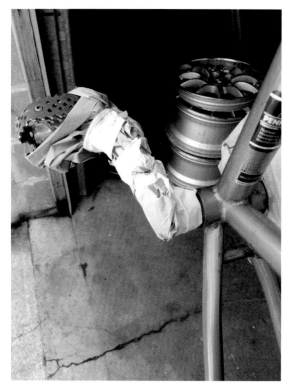

Figure 5-18 *Tape off the areas you don't want painted*

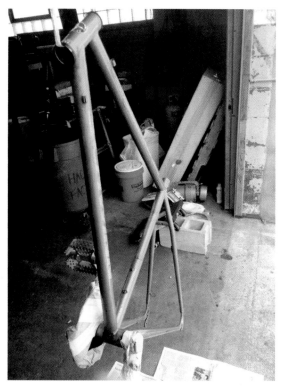

Figure 5-19 *Hang your bike up so the paint job looks good*

4. Hang your bike from a tree, rafter, or clothesline (as seen in Figure 5-19). Thread the line through a hollow part in the bike, like the head tube (if you removed the handlebars and fork) or a connector hole. This allows you to spray the frame, then let it dry, all without touching it.

5. You can now paint the bike. You may want to begin with a coat of primer. Once that is dry, spray on a coat of paint. Let the first coat dry for 24 hours, then give it at least one more coat. Finally, when you have the paint the way you like it, consider spraying a coat of clear enamel on the frame.

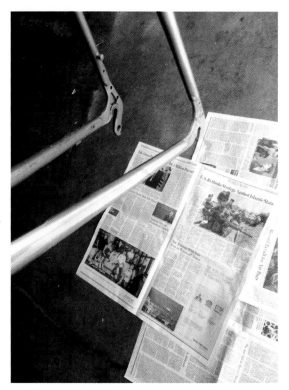

Figure 5-20 *It's time to paint your bike*

Project #6: Making a Fixie

Your freshly painted bike is incomplete—now is the time to replace the various moving parts, cables, reflectors, and anything else damaged during use. However, maybe you don't want to put it all back?

Fixies are bikes with no gear shifts, derailleurs, or brakes. If you want to stop, you either have to rely on your skill as a cyclist or else just put your foot down! Fixies are not for everyone, but if you do want to fixie-fy your bike, it's not too difficult. Assuming you're starting with a stripped down bike, here's how:

1. Make sure you have the right rear dropout. You want the kind that has a horizontal slot, not a vertical one (Figure 5-21). This gives you the ability to tension the chain by moving the rear wheel closer or farther away. Ordinarily,

the rear derailleur is adjusted to give the chain the right amount of tension.

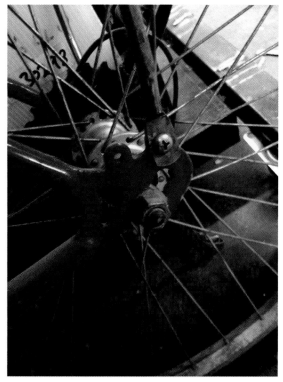

Figure 5-21 *Make sure you have this kind of dropout*

If you don't have the right kind of frame, it's still possible to make your bike a fixie. You'll have to buy or make horizontal dropouts, cut off the old dropouts, and weld on the new ones. You can learn how to do that sort of thing in Chapter 7.

2. You'll need to get the right kind of rear wheel. Unlike multispeed bikes, rear wheels on fixies don't have freewheels and cassettes. All they should have is a single-speed cog, often called a fixie cog, shown in Figure 5-22. A wheel designed to have a freewheel is different. Some people try to convert a freewheel into a fixed wheel bike by supergluing the freewheel mechanism, but

you're better off getting a new wheel and putting a fixie cog on it.

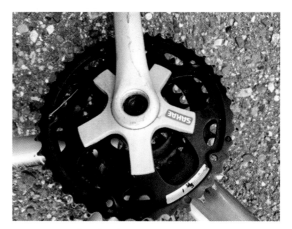

Figure 5-23 *Put the chain on the chainring, and either remove or ignore the forward cassette*

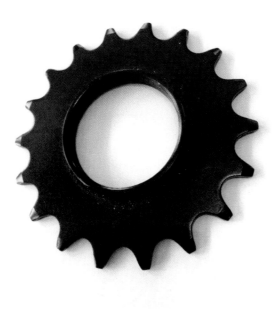

Figure 5-22 *A fixie cog takes the place of the gear cassette and freewheel*

3. You may be able to simply remove the front cassette with your cone wrench and use the chainring as the forward cog. On the other hand, it's easy to simply ignore the cassette—it simply won't get used (Figure 5-23).

However, some people buy specialized fixed-gear chainrings that offer different tooth configurations to help fixie riders get the gear ratios they're looking for.

4. Now you'll need to modify the chain. You will almost certainly have to remove some of the links (Figure 5-24) because the chain was long enough to be manipulated by the rear derailleur. You do this by using your chain breaker (mentioned in Chapter 4) to remove the pin from one link, then another a few links apart, then joining the now-shorter chain by inserting a pin with the chain breaker. Even with links removed, you will have to adjust the wheel's position in the dropout to properly tension the chain.

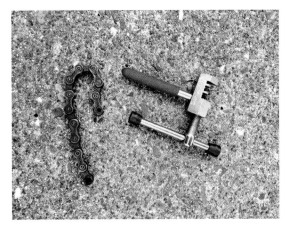

Figure 5-24 *You'll have to adjust the chain size*

5. Finally, you need to replace the front wheel, the seat, and the rest of the bike. Leave off reattaching the gear shifts, because you don't need them! As far as brakes go, that is a little more complicated. Premade fixies often have coaster brakes, but failing that, most bike riders would like to have a single brake for the rear wheel. Other, crazier cyclists skip the brakes altogether, trusting in their ability to slow the bike down simply by controlling how fast the pedals turn. Basically, if you want to slow down, pedal slower! If you're going to go this route, good luck!

Summary

In this chapter, you got your hands dirty (hopefully literally) by stripping down your bike, repainting it, and then rebuilding it as a fixie. In Chapter 6, you'll continue your exploration by tackling (wait for it!) wheels in all their variations and configurations.

All About Wheels

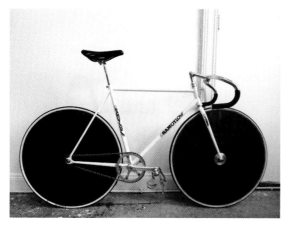

Wheels are arguably the most important part of a bike, and some of them are pretty crazy, like the Kevlar ones shown in Figure 6-1.

Figure 6-1 *This racing bike sports spokeless wheels built out of Kevlar (Photo credit: Sir Braginski)*

Rather than go the crazy route, however, this chapter explores such practical topics as the different types of wheels you're likely to encounter on the street. You'll also have an opportunity to master a number of critical maintenance tasks involving wheels: fixing a flat, properly inflating a tire, replacing a spoke, and removing wheels from the bike frame.

Anatomy of the Wheel

What's the difference between a tire and a wheel? The two terms are often conflated. The wheel usually refers to the entire assembly, while a tire is one of the (usually rubber, usually inflatable) components that go into it. Let's learn the parts of the typical bike wheel, following along with Figure 6-2:

1. Tube (not visible because it's inside the tire!)
2. Tire
3. Valve
4. Rim
5. Nipple
6. Reflector
7. Spokes
8. Hub
9. Hub shell
10. Cassette
11. Quick release

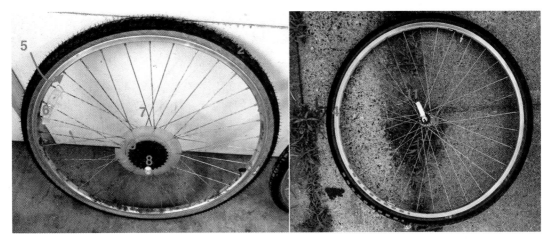

Figure 6-2 *A typical wheel*

Wheel Dimensions

For a long time, each manufacturer built its own wheels, and they were all different. In this age of international standards, the range of sizes has settled down into a few commonplace ones. ISO 5775 suggests the following dimensions.

Road/Racing Wheel

The ISO standard 622mm/29" wheel is the most common style of wheel in the US, used for most nonspecialty bicycles. It's called the 700C because the diameter is closer to 700mm with a stock tire on the rim; the diameter is measured from the outside edge of the rubber.

Mountain Bike Wheel

These wheels are built tougher than touring wheels, with heavier and sometimes wider rims. They're typically smaller, closer to 26 inches, and the standard is called 600C. However, a popular "29" rim is available.

BMX

These wheels are smaller: 20 inches in diameter, or 406mm. They're built smaller than racing and touring bikes because they're often used in kids' bikes. They're also built very robustly for their size, with some BMX bikes even having plastic bars in place of spokes, adding to the weight but making the wheel more durable.

Wheel Maintenance

In this section, we'll cover a number of critical skills necessary to keep your wheels rolling. First, you'll learn how to fix a flat tire on the road, using only a mini toolkit. After that, I'll show you the right way to inflate a tire. Finally, sometimes your wheels aren't aligned, and I'll show you how to true your wheels.

Fixing a Flat

You're riding along and suddenly a tire goes flat. What do you do? Well, if you have the on-the-go toolkit I showed you in Chapter 4, you're in business!

1. Remove the wheel, as shown in Figure 6-3. If the front wheel was punctured, this is a very easy step—all you have to do is hit a quick release or turn a hex bolt with your multitool. If it's the rear wheel, follow these substeps:

    a. Shift to the smallest gears, making the chain as loose as possible.

b. Open the brake by releasing the cable that controls it.

c. Pull back the derailleur and chain to get it out of the way.

d. Unbolt the rear wheel and remove it.

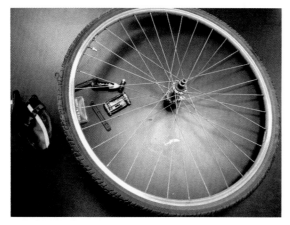

Figure 6-3 *Remove the wheel with the flat tire*

2. Deflate the tire the rest of the way, then use a tire lever to pull the wheel away from the rim, as seen in Figure 6-4. You may need multiple levers if the rubber is especially stiff.

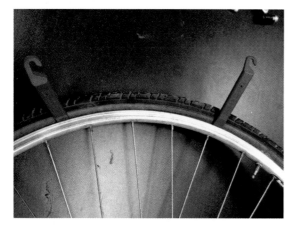

Figure 6-4 *Tire levers pull the tire away from the rim*

3. Pull out the inner tube and locate the puncture, as seen in Figure 6-5.

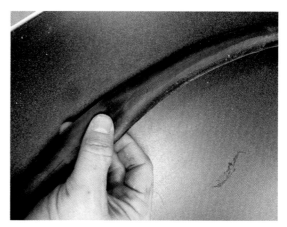

Figure 6-5 *Inspect the inner tube for punctures*

4. Score the rubber around the puncture (Figure 6-6) using the rasp from your tire repair kit.

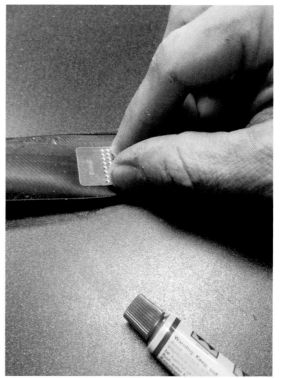

Figure 6-6 *Roughen the area around the puncture*

5. Apply glue around the puncture and add a patch, as seen in Figure 6-7.

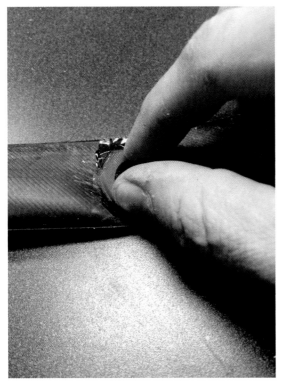

Figure 6-7 *Glue and patch*

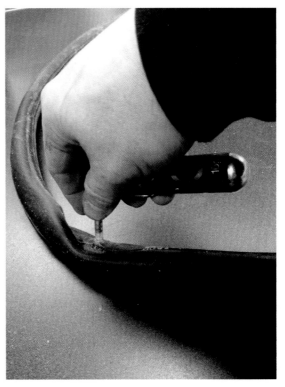

Figure 6-8 *Fill up the tire partially*

6. Use just a puff from your CO2 cartridge (Figure 6-8) to refill the inner tube partially, so that it holds its shape but still fits readily into the tire.

7. Insert the tube in the tire, then reattach it to the rim, popping the tire lip back under the edge of the rim, as shown in Figure 6-9. Don't use your tire levers to put the tube back in, because they can puncture the tube.

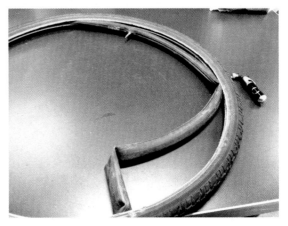

Figure 6-9 *Pop the tire back under the rim*

8. Finish inflating the tire, then reattach the wheel (Figure 6-10). You're rolling!

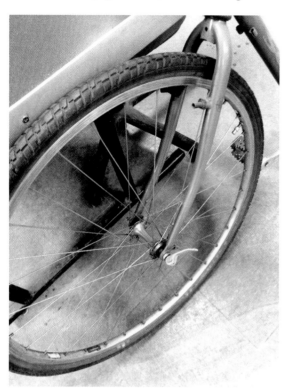

Figure 6-10 *Put the wheel back on*

Inflating a Tire

A properly inflated tire reduces the friction between wheel and road, making your ride easier while preserving the wheel's rubber tread.

Here is the correct way to inflate your bicycle's tires:

1. Find the PSI (pounds per square inch) rating for the wheel. Usually it's printed in raised letters on the side of the wheel.

2. Open the valve.

3. Inflate in short bursts, especially if you're using a compressor.

4. Pause periodically to test the PSI with your pressure gauge (Figure 6-11).

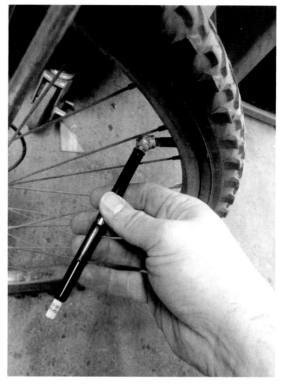

Figure 6-11 *Measure the PSI to make sure you're properly inflated*

Tightening or Replacing a Spoke

Spokes typically are attached at the hub with a simple loop, and at the rim with tapered nuts called nipples. Use the spoke wrench I mentioned in Chapter 4 to tighten or loosen the spokes (Figure 6-12). In addition to being able to replace a spoke that is damaged, you could use this technique to adjust the length of the spoke, which changes the angle of the rim in comparison to the hub. Nipples are counterthreaded, so you'll have to turn them clockwise to loosen.

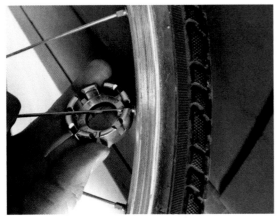

Figure 6-12 *Tighten the nipple using your spoke wrench*

Truing a Wheel

Another use for this spoke-adjusting technique is to ensure the wheel runs smoothly by selectively adjusting its spokes. This is called truing. Here's how you do it:

1. Suspend the bike (preferably in a bike mechanic's stand). The wheels will need to rotate smoothly.

2. Rotate the tire while looking at the space between the bike wheel and the brake pads. Ideally that space shouldn't be changing, but if the wheel is out of true, it will seem to wobble.

3. Where it seems particularly far from the pad (Figure 6-13), tighten the spoke on that side. This will pull the rim over somewhat to even it out.

4. Repeat until you can't spot any obvious wobbling. You're trued!

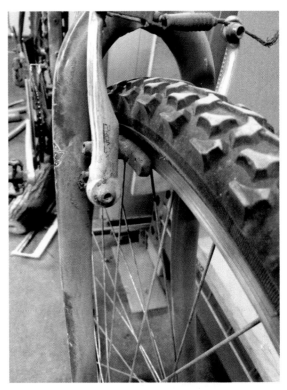

Figure 6-13 *Watch the space between the rim and the brake pad*

Summary

You learned about wheels in this chapter, covering the dimensions of standard-sized wheels, as well as some basic techniques for maintaining them. Now it's time to tackle frames! In Chapter 7, you'll learn how to weld up your own frame, and how to hack and modify an existing frame.

Hacking Frames 7

Expensive frames aren't necessarily better. They may have more graceful curves, or prettier paint. Some use carbon fiber or another advanced material, thereby justifying the cost, but many are just welded steel. In this chapter, you'll continue your metal mastery by learning how to hack your own frame. You'll work on two projects: first, you'll assemble a frame using new steel tubes and gaskets, as seen in Figure 7-1.

Then, you'll further use your skills when you "chop" a bike by modifying its frame. There could be a practical reason for this, or maybe you'll just want to put a nonstandard curve on the tubes to make it look a little cooler. Either way, you'll learn a lot about working with metal.

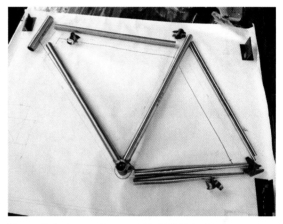

Figure 7-1 *A partially assembled DIY bike frame*

Parts of a Frame

Let's delve deeper into the parts of the frame, following along with Figure 7-2:

1. Bottom bracket: The crankset connects to this bracket, and it serves as sort of a hub for four tubes.

2. Chain stays: These lightweight tubes connect from the bottom bracket to the rear wheel's dropouts.

3. Down tube: The slanting tube at the front of the bike, leading from the head tube to the bottom bracket.

4. Dropouts: The rear wheel connects to these dropouts, which are supported by the chain stays and the seat stays.

5. Fork: This is where the front wheel is installed.

6. Head tube: The tube through which the fork passes.

7. Top tube: The main horizontal tube of the frame.

8. Seat stays: Slender tubes that help support the rear wheel.

9. Seat tube: The vertical tube in a bike frame into which the seat is mounted.

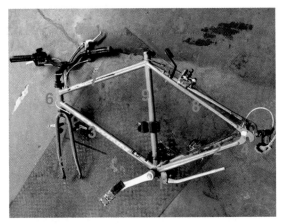

Figure 7-2 *Every tube on a bike has a name*

How to Weld and Braze

Welding and brazing are both great ways to join a bike frame's tubes together. Brazing is a technique, similar to soldering, that uses a low-melting brass or bronze filler, called braze, to attach two pieces of metal together, rather than actually melting the two parts. By contrast, welding involves melting the actual steel, while applying additional metal in the form of a welding rod.

Procedure

The following steps show you how to braze. Just be aware that working with metal can be messy, expensive, and potentially dangerous if you don't know what you're doing. When first learning, you should always have a buddy with prior brazing experience guiding you through the process. I also recommend watching YouTube videos describing the tools and walking through using them in an actual project. It's a great way to bone up before you work on your frame.

These are the steps you should follow:

1. First, you need to clean all surfaces. A joint that is sticking to dirt and dust won't be as secure as one that attaches metal-to-metal, so be sure to clean all surfaces using ordinary all-purpose cleaning spray and paper towels, as seen in Figure 7-3. Similarly, you won't want to braze painted metal, so sand or file off any leftover paint. Console yourself in knowing you're going to have to repaint the bike anyway!

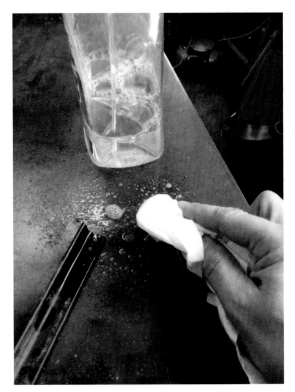

Figure 7-3 *Clean all surfaces thoroughly*

2. Inspect the fit between the various parts (Figure 7-4) to ensure that there isn't too much or too little gap between them. The braze must flow between the parts to stick them together, so they actually shouldn't have a 100% perfect fit. Use your hacksaw and files to shape the ends as needed. At the same time, you don't want the braze to be bridging too much of a gap, so don't take out too much material—aim for a hair's-width gap.

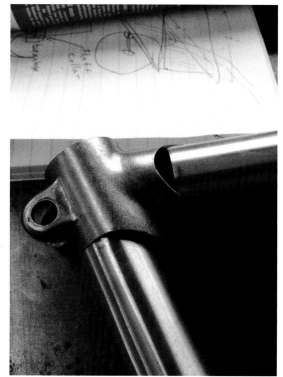

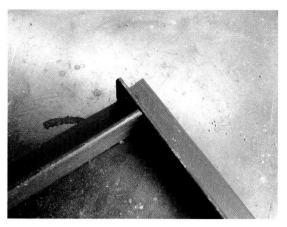

Figure 7-4 *Check the fit between the various parts*

3. Optionally, you can insert lugs, gussets, or other support material. Lugs help secure the hollow ends of the tube, and they can be brazed into place just like any other part. Figure 7-5 shows a lug being placed.

Figure 7-5 *Lugs help you join two metal tubes*

4. You can now apply flux (if necessary). Flux is a substance that helps molten metal flow more readily, and facilitates the joining of two dissimilar surfaces. I used brazing rods with flux already coating them (Figure 7-6), but if you are just using bare wire for the brazing material, you'll need a separate flux. Dip a warm piece of brazing rod into the open tin of flux to coat the rod.

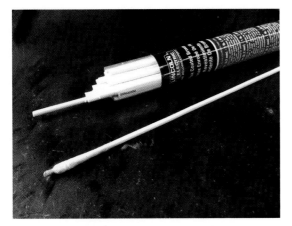

Figure 7-6 *These brazing rods come pre-fluxed*

5. Next, you need to steady the parts to be joined. Clamp at least one of the two parts, with the other one held in your nondominant hand, while your primary hand holds the torch. Better yet would be to use a series of clamps, as shown in Figure 7-7, to hold everything in place while you work.

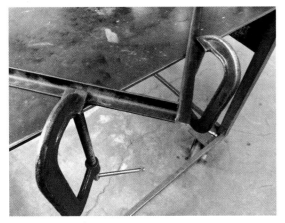

Figure 7-7 *Hold the parts in position so they can be brazed*

6. Use your torch to heat up the join to be brazed, then apply the tip of your brazing rod, allowing the filler metal to flow into the gap (Figure 7-8).

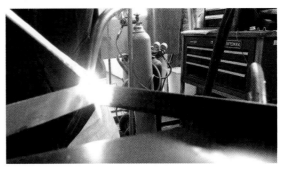

Figure 7-8 *Apply braze to the heated join*

7. Finally, you need to clean up: use a grinder to polish off the excess metal (Figure 7-9).

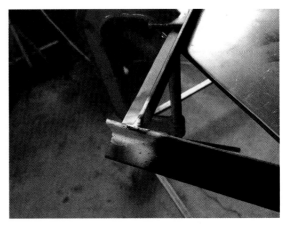

Figure 7-9 *Clean all surfaces thoroughly*

Project #7: Braze Up a Frame

Now you're ready to build your own frame (Figure 7-10)! This is a great exercise that will help you build the perfect bicycle for you: one that is functionally yours, sized perfectly for your body, and configured exactly the way you want it. There's also the pride in knowing that you built your own bike. Finally, creating your own frame also gives you the opportunity to make the bike unique in appearance. Your bike doesn't have to be the same as the ones at the store!

Let's get started.

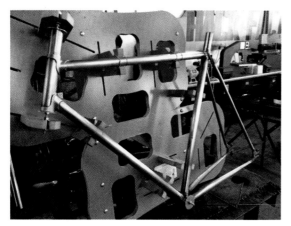

Figure 7-10 *Let's braze up a frame!*

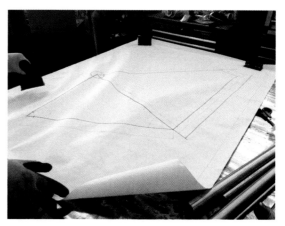

Figure 7-11 *Design your frame at 1:1 scale*

Parts List

You'll need the following parts to build a frame:

- Set of pipes
- Set of lugs
- Brazing rod
- Flux
- Oxy-acetylene torch
- Clamps
- Hacksaw
- Files

Procedure

Once you've collected the parts and materials you need, you can begin building the bike frame of your dreams. These are the steps you'll need to follow.

1. First, you need to design your frame. What size tubes will you use? At what angles will they be positioned? Sometimes it's helpful to draw out the design at full size, using a big piece of paper (Figure 7-11) so you can see how it will look.

2. Measure the angles for the pipes, using your design, as shown in Figure 7-12.

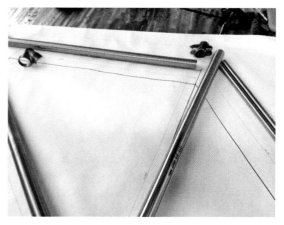

Figure 7-12 *Measure angles to ensure a proper fit*

3. Use a hacksaw to cut into the pipes so they fit together reasonably well—it's not the Space Shuttle, but you don't want there to be too much gap for the braze to bridge. Figure 7-13 shows how it should look.

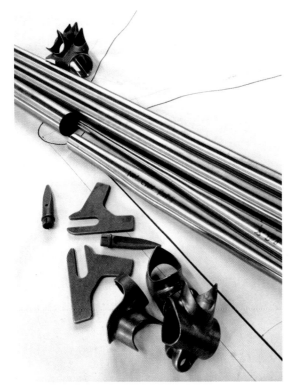

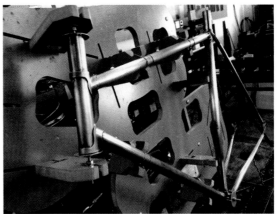

Figure 7-14 *Secure the tubes for welding*

5. Connect the correct lugs (seen in Figure 7-15) to your bike's head tube, insert the top and down tubes, then braze them up.

Figure 7-13 *Cut the tubes so they fit together*

The preceding three steps assume you aren't buying a kit with preconfigured lugs and tubes. But if you are using a kit, you may find you don't have to do those three steps, as they will likely have been done for you already.

---

4. Next, you'll want to secure the tubes so you can weld them up. You *could* weld them up one at a time, but likely the angles would be all over the place. Ideally all the tubes should be clamped at the same time. One way is to make or buy a frame-welding jig, like the Jiggernaut (*http://www.flatpackfoundry.com*), shown in Figure 7-14. It's a great way to make a professional-looking bike in your own garage.

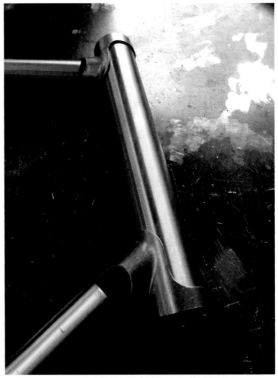

Figure 7-15 *Braze the tubes together with the help of some lugs*

6. Next, you'll secure the bottom bracket (Figure 7-16). This is a very complicated

part and it's imperative that you don't get anything on the threads inside the bracket. It's also easy to push the tubes in too far—be sure to keep the ends clear of the main threaded area inside.

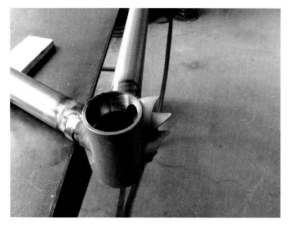

Figure 7-16 *Braze up the bottom bracket*

7. Braze the seat tube to the bottom bracket and top tube, as seen in Figure 7-17.

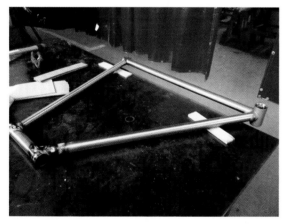

Figure 7-17 *Attach the seat tube to the bottom bracket and top tube*

8. Next, let's work on the seat stays. These get lugs brazed to them, as seen in Figure 7-18.

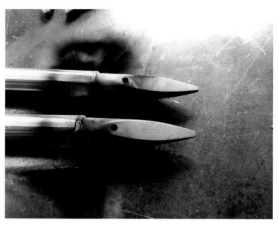

Figure 7-18 *Attach two lugs to the seat stays*

9. At this point, you need to cut the stays (as necessary). Some dropouts have plugs built into them, but the ones shown in Figure 7-19 do not. If that's the case, you'll have to use a bandsaw or hacksaw to cut slits in the tubes so they'll fit on the dropouts.

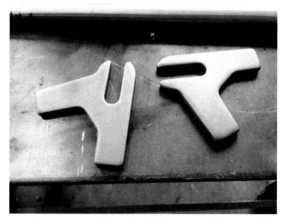

Figure 7-19 *Cut slits in the stays to accommodate the dropouts*

10. Braze the un-slit ends of the seat stays to the appropriate lugs built into the bottom bracket (Figure 7-20).

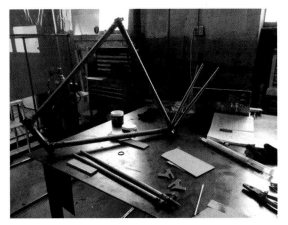

Figure 7-20 *Braze the chain stays to the bottom bracket*

11. All four stays get brazed to the two dropouts, with each dropout getting one seat and one chain stay. Figure 7-21 shows how it should look.

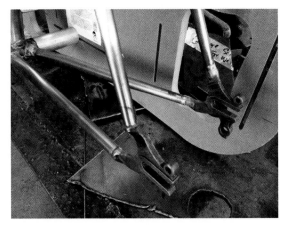

Figure 7-21 *Braze on the dropouts*

12. The last part of the main frame build consists of brazing the pointy lugs of the seat stays (seen in Figure 7-22) to the seat tube.

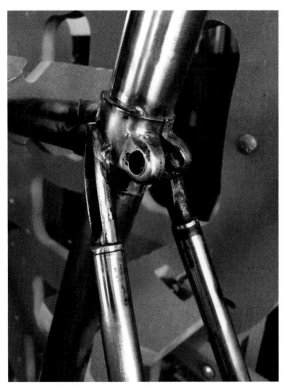

Figure 7-22 *Braze the pointy lugs to the seat tube (Photo credit: Gabriel Amadeus, Creative Commons)*

Make a Chopper

Maybe you don't want to go to all the trouble —and let's face it, expense—to weld up your own frame when there are a million scrap bikes floating around. Grab one of those cheapies and make it your own by chopping it! Figure 7-23 shows an example of combining two bikes.

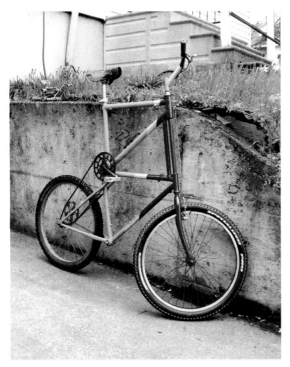

Figure 7-23 *Don't like your bike? Just add another bike. (Photo credit: Gabriel Amadeus, Creative Commons)*

1. You'll need to strip down the bike, following the same steps you did in this chapter's "Procedure". You should focus on removing parts and paint anywhere close to where you'll be cutting or brazing.

2. Just hack it! I mean that in the hacksaw sense. Now is the time to saw through tubes you want to modify. Most bikes are just steel, making them relatively easy to cut through.

3. Arrange two half-frames together so you can get a sense of how it will look when assembled. It's not a bad idea to double-check that your chain and brake cables will still work when you get everything back together!

4. You might want to look into buying lugs, such as you used when you welded up your frame—these may be purchased in a variety of configurations. However, lugs aren't necessary. If you're able to fit the tube-ends together snugly, simply weld or braze from there.

5. Follow the welding directions I gave earlier in the chapter. You'll especially want to clean the paint off the hacked sections of frame.

Summary

In this chapter, you brazed up your own frame and also made a chopper. This is important stuff to learn, because it allows you to modify the bones of the bike to make it work better for you, or simply to add uniqueness. In Chapter 8, you'll focus on adding electronics to your bike, beginning with the all-important power supply.

Adding Power

Enough with the metal—let's check out how to add electronics to our bikes. In this chapter, you'll explore what it takes to provide electrical power for your bike. First, you'll add a solar cell, which allows you to charge your phone while you ride. Then, I'll show you how to attach a weatherproof enclosure, which can hold a battery pack and microcontroller, to your bike. This will prepare you for later chapters, which include progressively more complicated electronics projects.

First, however, you're going to learn an important skill necessary for building electronics projects: soldering. Read on!

Project #8: How to Solder (the Quick Version)

The following is a very quick guide to learning to solder.

Soldering has a lot in common with brazing, which you learned in Chapter 7. In both cases, you use a filler material with a low melting point to bind to components with high melting points. Solder is usually a mixture of lead and tin, and it conducts electricity, allowing you to construct permanent circuits with wires, components, and chips.

Not surprisingly, soldering is also much cheaper than welding to learn and perform. Soldering essentially consists of putting components on a printed circuit board (PCB) and attaching them to each other in the right way with a conductive metal (solder). You don't need tanks of flammable gas and a welding torch to do soldering; you only need a handheld, electrically powered heating element called a soldering iron to stick everything together.

Parts List

The tools pictured in Figure 8-1 are part of a simplified learn-to-solder kit, sold as the Make:it Soldering Starter Kit (*http://bit.ly/1LQi9sl*) (P/N MKRAD04) in the Maker Shed. Here's what you get:

- Soldering iron: This is a basic model with one temperature setting. This is OK, because most beginners just use one setting anyway. If you want a fancier iron with an adjustable temperature, I suggest the Weller WES-51. I've used one for several years and swear by it. Jameco.com is one of many sites that sell it (P/N 217461).

- Extra soldering iron tips: After a while, soldering irons need new tips, and the Starter Kit includes a couple.

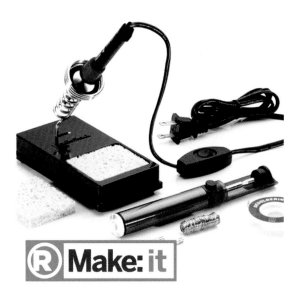

Figure 8-1 *You get these tools as part of the Make:it Soldering Starter Kit*

- Soldering stand: Your hot iron needs a place to rest when it's not in your hand. The soldering stand has a sponge that helps clean the iron's tip. Another tool people often use in place of the sponge is a tangle of brass shavings called a "brass sponge" (a good one is Adafruit, P/N 1172). It helps keep the tip clean, but without water.

- Solder: This solder has a core of rosin, which acts as flux so you don't need to flux up your parts prior to soldering. I usually recommend 60% tin/40% lead, 0.5mm, rosin-core lead solder, available from Adafruit.com (P/N 1886) and most other electronics stores.

- Solder sucker: You use this to desolder —sucking out molten solder if you put too much in, or to remove a part from the circuit board.

- Desoldering braid: When the solder sucker won't get that last piece of solder, this braid might do the trick, wicking it up like a paper towel tackles a spill.

- Wire cutter/stripper: This isn't actually in the kit, which is why it's not shown here. I suggest a nice pair of Hakko cutters available from SparkFun (P/N 12630).

Procedure

Follow along with these steps to solder:

1. Set up your soldering area. Some sort of clamp like a "helping hand" tool (e.g., Maker Shed, P/N MKHH1) or desk vise (e.g., Maker Shed, P/N MKPV02) works great to hold the circuit board in place. You'll also want your iron, clippers, and extra solder close at hand. You can see a sample setup in Figure 8-2.

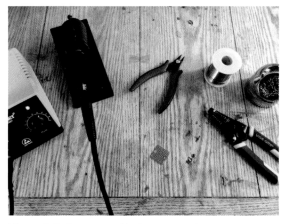

Figure 8-2 *Get your soldering area ready to go*

2. Make sure your iron is hot. Some irons have only a single temperature setting, while others are adjustable. I usually keep my iron set at 650°F, and this is good for most uses. When the iron is hot, coat the tip of the iron with a thin layer of solder (Figure 8-3). Called tinning, this helps the iron to conduct temperature more efficiently, and makes for superior soldering.

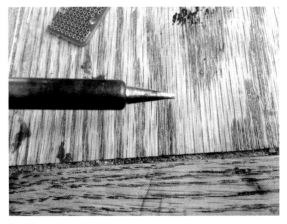

Figure 8-3 *Tin the tip of your soldering iron*

3. Connect the parts you wish to solder. Most hobbyist kits use through-hole components, which consist of an electronic component with wires (leads) coming out of them. You slide the leads through solder pads on the circuit board, and solder the leads into place. One common tactic is to bend back one of the leads so the part doesn't come out. You can see an example of this in Figure 8-4.

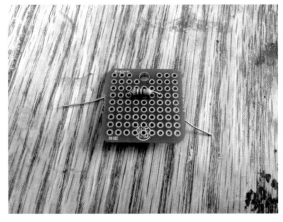

Figure 8-4 *Bend back to the leads from behind, then solder*

4. Solder it up! Once you have the part's leads inserted into the holes, flip over the board and solder in the part from *underneath*. This is how you do it:

touch the hot tip of the soldering iron to both the component's lead and the solder pad, as shown in Figure 8-5. After a couple of seconds, touch a length of solder to the two surfaces and a neat little hill of solder should flow into place. Remember, the point is not to melt the solder directly with the soldering iron. It to use the soldering iron to heat the components, and let *them* melt the solder around them.

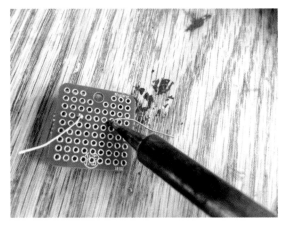

Figure 8-5 *Touch the iron's tip to both the pad and the lead*

5. Clip the leads. The excess wire from the component is still sticking out from the PCB. Use your wire cutters to snip the leads close to the PCB. It helps to hold your hand over the board as a kind of shield, as a snipped component wire can go flying through the air and hit someone in the eye. The end result of snipping the wire should look just like Figure 8-6.

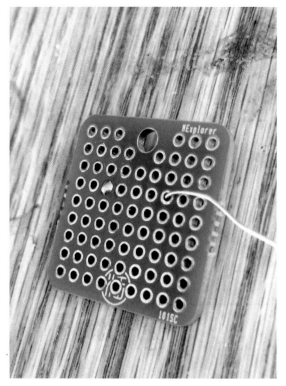

Figure 8-6 *You're done!*

Cleanup and Lead Concerns

Solder is made of tin and lead, and lead is poisonous. So, how do you use it safely? The good news is that as long as you don't eat any lead chips, you'll probably be OK. Just follow these simple guidelines:

- When soldering, don't touch your face with your hands after you've touched solder. It'd be as if you were hanging out with someone with a cold. Just wash your hands before you do *anything* besides solder.

- When you're done, wipe down the work surface using all-purpose cleaner spray and paper towels. Make sure to snag any glops of solder that fell off. Clean off your tools to make sure they don't have any lead residue.

See? Basic cleanliness is really all it takes to use solder safely.

Harnessing Solar Power

Now that you're ready to solder, let's tackle our first electronic project.

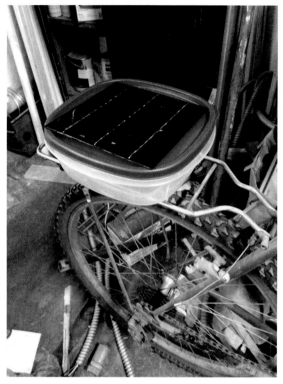

Figure 8-7 *Build this solar-powered battery pack*

The solar charger project shows how to build a sun-powered battery pack for your bike (Figure 8-7). This will let you charge your phone or power a project, all without having to rely on battery or generated power. It's an easy and useful project that will put you in the mood for hacking more electronics onto your bike!

Parts List

Gather together the following parts:

- Solar panel (Adafruit, P/N 417): This panel generates 6 volts at 3.7 watts in direct sunlight.

- LiOn charger (Adafruit, P/N 390): This charger regulates the output of the solar cell, converting it to a steady 5V.

- PowerBoost 500 (Adafruit, P/N 1903): This module keeps the voltage at the correct levels so that a smartphone will take the charge.

- Battery (Adafruit, P/N 1578): A LiOn rated at 3.7V 500mAh worked well for me.

- USB-A female breakout board (SparkFun P/N 12700): This board has a USB-A socket and breaks down USB's four wires into separate pins.

- Male DC power adapter (Adafruit, P/N 369): This converts a barrel-jack power coupling, such as is found on the LiOn charger, into regular wires via screw-terminals.

- 7" plastic sandwich box: You can find these at your local grocery store (they're most often associated with brown-bag lunch technology). However, in this project, it will serve as a waterproof enclosure. The one I used was a Rubbermaid 9-cup.

- Double-sided tape or hot glue

Procedure

Follow along with these steps to build your solar charger:

1. Drill holes in your sandwich container (Figure 8-8); they should be the same size and spacing as the wires attached to your solar panel. Don't make the holes any bigger than they need to be —they're just going to have to be sealed later, and a smaller hole is a more successfully sealed hole.

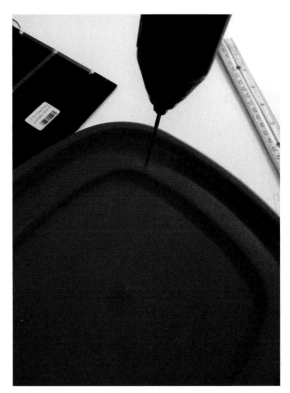

Figure 8-8 *Drill holes in the sandwich box with identical spacing as the solar panel's wires*

2. Thread the solar panel's wires through the holes you just drilled. Attach the DC power adapter's screw terminals to the wires, as shown in Figure 8-9. This allows you to plug the output of the solar panel directly into the LiOn charger.

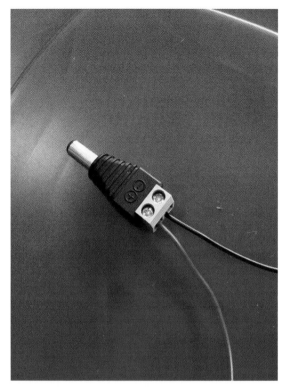

Figure 8-9 *Attach the DC power adapter to the solar panel's wires*

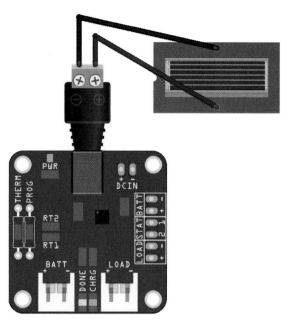

Figure 8-10 *Connect the power adapter to the battery charger*

3. Connect the power adapter to the barrel plug on the LiOn charger, as shown in Figure 8-10.

4. Solder a red wire to the hole marked "VCC" on the USB breakout board. Solder the black wire to the hole marked "GND". It should look just like Figure 8-11.

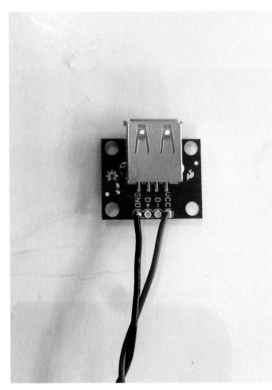

Figure 8-11 *Solder the red and black wires*

5. Add the PowerBoost module. If we had a battery like a LiPo feeding the Power-Boost, it would plug into the JST connector. However, because we're just using wires, you should solder in red and black wires as you see in Figure 8-12,

with the positive lead on LOAD connecting to VCC on the PowerBoost (shown as a red wire), and the negative lead (black) soldered into GND.

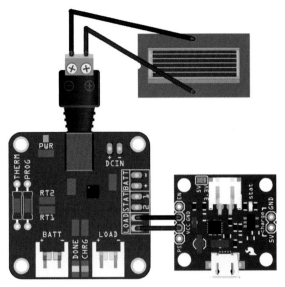

Figure 8-12 *Connect the PowerBoost module*

6. Solder in the wires from the USB breakout board. The red wire connects to the 5V pin on the PowerBoost, and the black wire plugs into GND, as shown in Figure 8-13. While you're at it, plug in your favorite USB cable to the matching port on the breakout board.

Harnessing Solar Power

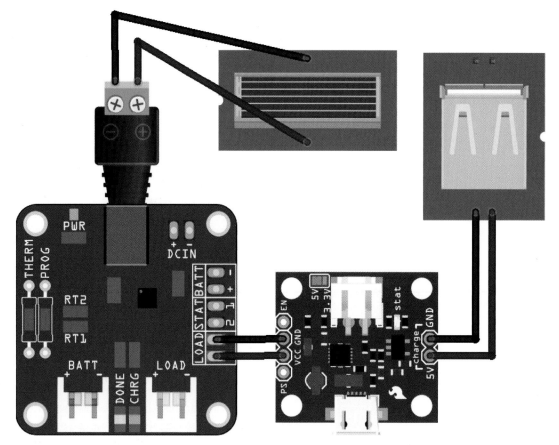

Figure 8-13 *Solder in the USB breakout*

7. Add the battery. This plugs into the BATT port on the LiPo charger, as shown in Figure 8-14. The solar cell will charge the battery, so that if a cloud covers the sun, your phone will continue to charge without a hitch, as it will be drawing its power from the battery!

74   Make: Bicycle Projects

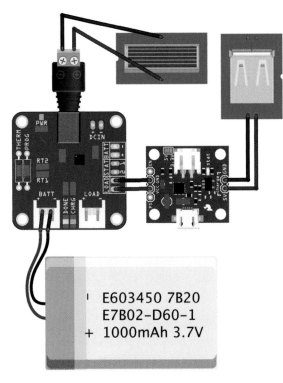

Figure 8-14 *Plug in the battery*

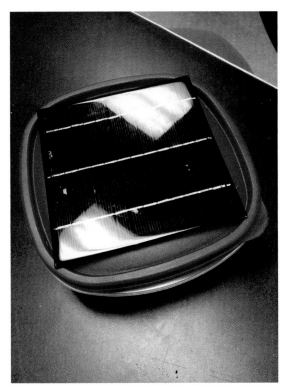

Figure 8-15 *Attach the solar panel to the lid of the box*

8. Using double-sided tape or hot glue, attach the solar panel to the lid of the plastic box (Figure 8-15), and place all the other components inside. You may want to seal up the wire-holes from the inside as well, using more hot glue. The solar panel is encased in clear plastic, so it is weatherproof, but the charger and other electronics aren't protected. That's what the box is for!

9. Attach the completed solar charger to your bike. Simply zip-tying the assembly to your bike rack (Figure 8-16) is one way that works. Another option might be to attach it horizontally to the side of your bike, if you think that would get you better rays.

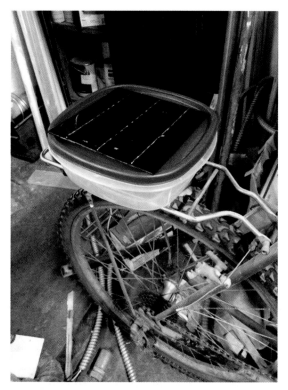

Figure 8-16 *Add the charger to your bike*

In order to charge your phone on the go, simply put the device in the sandwich box along with the electronics. You also have the option to attach the USB breakout board in a way that allows you to plug in your charging cable from *outside* the box. The breakout board has mounting holes so you can screw it to the box close to the edge. One big problem with this is that it breaks the weatherproofing on the sandwich box. You can glop it up with hot glue, but it will never be quite as sealed as before.

Add a Waterproof Microcontroller Pack

Here's another approach: let's skip the solar panel and just rely on battery power, allowing us to have a much smaller package—those solar panels are big! And because we're saving space, we'll be able to fit a microcontroller into the waterproof enclosure as well. The controller we're using is an Arduino Uno, pretty much the

most popular and easiest-to-use board out there. Rather than relying on a sandwich box for an enclosure, you'll use a super-robust Pelican case (Figure 8-17) that is not only waterproof, but practically uncrushable.

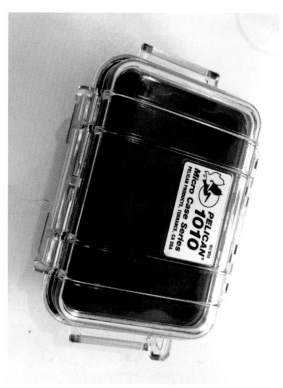

Figure 8-17 *This Pelican case makes a great Arduino enclosure*

Parts List

Gather together the following parts to build your microcontroller pack:

- Arduino Uno (Maker Shed, P/N MKSP99): This is the default Arduino and you can't go wrong with it.

- 9V battery and cable (Adafruit P/N 80): This cable has a barrel plug on one end and 9V snaps on the other.

- Pelican 1010 case: This box is water-resistant, practically indestructible, and just barely big enough for an Arduino and battery.

Procedure

To build your microcontroller pack, follow these steps:

1. Connect the battery to the battery cable (Figure 8-18), simply by snapping it into place.

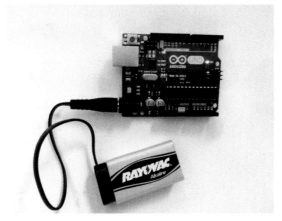

Figure 8-19 *Plug the power adapter into the Arduino*

3. Put the Arduino and battery in the case, as shown in Figure 8-20. You may want to use double-sided tape to keep the parts from bouncing around. Alternatively, you can drill mounting holes in the bottom of the Pelican case and more securely attach them together. This presents a slight problem: how do you keep the case waterproof? Because the holes are on the bottom of the case, and thereby protected from direct rain, a dab of hot glue on each screwhead should do the trick.

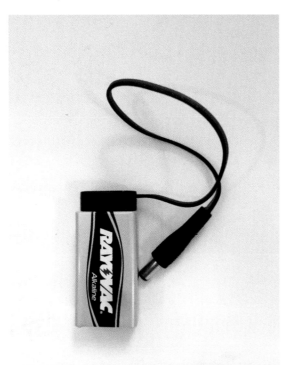

Figure 8-18 *The battery plugs into the cable*

2. Plug the power adapter's plug into the barrel connector on the Arduino. Figure 8-19 shows how it should look.

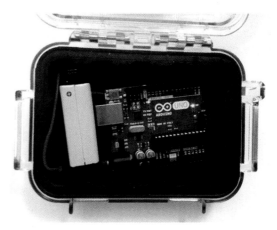

Figure 8-20 *Put the Arduino in the case*

4. Program the Arduino by popping open the case (Figure 8-21) and inserting the

usual USB cable. Of course you'll need to add sensors and other components if you want your Arduino to do anything! Don't worry, in upcoming chapters you'll do just that.

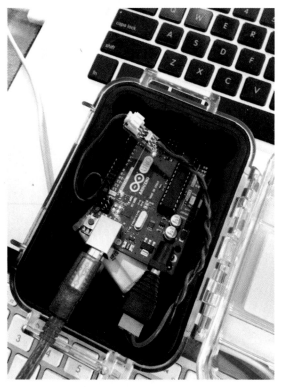

Figure 8-21 *Program your Arduino!*

Summary

Chapter 8 was all about powering your bike, with two different ways of powering bike-mounted projects. In Chapter 9, you'll put these projects to practical use by building a variety of projects based on light-emitting diodes (LEDs) that will make your bike look great!

Lighting It Up

This chapter shows readers how to build and install a couple of decorative LED projects, beginning with small, battery-powered lights I call Poesies. Then, we'll quickly ramp up the challenge with a DIY headlight that uses a high-brightness LED to illuminate the roadway ahead of you. The final project is an interactive LED strand (Figure 9-1) that responds to the bike's movements by altering the color and pattern of lights.

LED Poesies

The first light-up project is a fun little project that might be good for a kid's (or a whimsical adult's) bike. It's a big watch battery–powered LED that is part of a laser-cut wooden flower, seen in Figure 9-2. You can also riff on it to make more sophisticated displays as you get more confident with electronics. For now, it's just a very simple project to get you started.

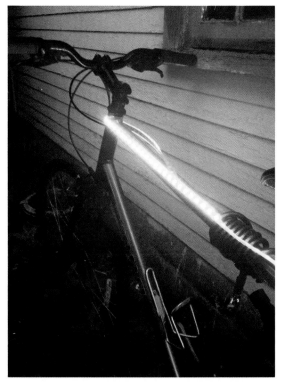

Figure 9-1 *You'll add this cool LED strip to your bike*

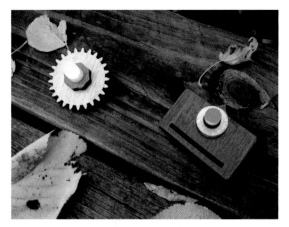

Figure 9-2 *Poesies are little light-up decorations*

Parts List

You need just a few parts to build an LED Poesy:

- Flower shape: I laser-cut fun shapes out of 3mm birch. You can download the shapes from my Thingiverse page (*http://www.thingiverse.com/jwb/designs*) or you can design your own.

- LED: I used a 10mm, color-changing LED (SparkFun, P/N 11452), but you can substitute a regular colored LED, like a red one from SparkFun (P/N 10632). You get the idea!

- Proto board: You'll need a printed circuit board (PCB) to stick everything to. I used a small section of stripboard (Mouser.com, P/N 854-ST1) but you could also use SparkFun's small square proto board, P/N 8808.

- Coin cell battery holder: SparkFun sells a good one (P/N 7948). You'll also need a matching battery, a CR1225 you can buy at many stores, including SparkFun (P/N 337).

- Switch: I used a SPDT switch from SparkFun (P/N 9609). SPDT stands for single pole, double throw. This means there is one circuit that can be controlled by the switch (the pole) and two positions or throws—those being on

and off. In other words, the most basic switch possible.

- Wire: You'll need just a small amount of wire. SparkFun sells a nice assortment of 22-gauge wire (P/N 11367). Or try your local electronics hobby store.

- Double-sided foam tape

Procedure

Follow these steps to create your LED Poesy:

1. Solder the battery clip to the proto board, as shown in Figure 9-3.

   You should make sure to leave the open end next to the edge of the board so you can put batteries in!

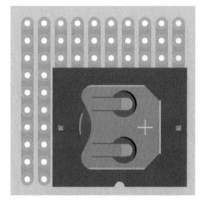

Figure 9-3 *Solder the battery clip*

2. Solder in the switch. You'll need to arrange the switch so that its three leads sit on three different buses of the stripboard. (Reminder: a bus is a whole strip of proto board that is electrically connected via strips of copper.) Figure 9-4 shows how it should look.

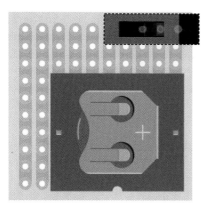

Figure 9-4 *Solder in the switch*

3. Wire the battery to the switch. The third lead of the switch (Figure 9-5) sits on the same bus as the positive lead of the battery holder. This is a clever way of saving a wire, but if you can't arrange your board this way, you'll need to solder a wire to connect those two components.

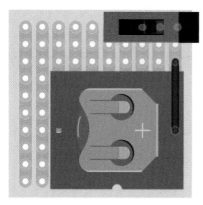

Figure 9-5 *Connect the battery to the switch*

4. Thread the leads of the LED through the holes in the wooden flower shape as well as the *back* of the stripboard, so that you're sandwiching the flower between the LED and the board. Figure 9-6 shows how it should look. Use double-sided tape to secure the board to the flower. Solder the leads into the stripboard, making sure to remember which lead was positive.

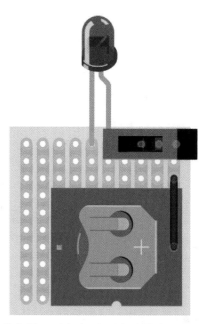

Figure 9-6 *Thread the leads of the LED through the wooden shape*

5. Solder a wire from the middle pole of the switch to the positive lead of the LED, shown as a purple wire in Figure 9-7.

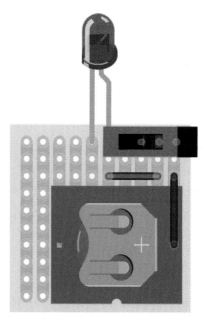

Figure 9-7 *Add a wire leading from the switch to the LED*

6. Solder a wire that connects the negative lead of the LED to the ground lead of the battery. You can see how it should look in Figure 9-8.

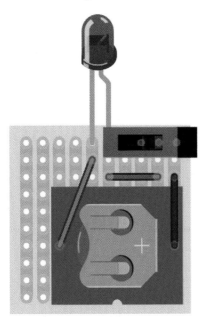

Figure 9-8 *Connect the negative lead of the LED to the battery's ground*

Project #9: Accelerometer-Controlled LED Strand

The next project is a little more sophisticated, and uses the Arduino enclosure you assembled in Chapter 8. It consists of a lovely strand of RGB LEDs (Figure 9-9) that change their color and pattern to conform to the movement of the bike.

On NeoPixels

The LED strand I used for this project is part of a line of RGB LEDs called NeoPixels, an example of which can be seen in Figure 9-9. These LEDs, sold by Adafruit, are great for projects like this because they have an LED control chip underneath every pixel, giving you an extraordinary amount of control over the strand with just a single data wire, in addition to the usual wires for power and ground.

NeoPixels are part of a larger category of LED called smart LEDs, and typically they allow you to change the brightness and color of any or all of the pixels at will—so long as they are plugged into a microcontroller, of course. While smart, NeoPixels still need a brain to guide them.

You can learn more about NeoPixel configurations (single LEDs, rings, strips, and matrices) and how to program them on Adafruit's website (*https://learn.adafruit.com/adafruit-neopixel-uberguide*).

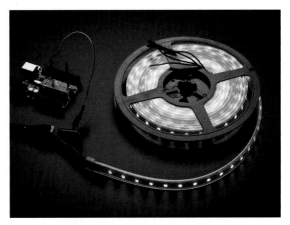

Figure 9-9 *NeoPixels are a great line of smart LEDs (Photo credit: Adafruit Industries)*

Parts List

In addition to the Arduino, battery, and Pelican case specified in the project in Chapter 8, you'll need the following:

- Adafruit Perma-Proto board: This is a solderable prototyping board (Maker Shed, P/N MKAD48) designed for projects that you want to keep around after you build. They're more durable than a solderless breadboard (Maker Shed, P/N MKKN2) but also make it harder to fix if you mess up.

- NeoPixel LED Strip: Adafruit sells a 60-LED NeoPixel strip (P/N 1461) that you'll use to decorate your bike.

- 1000uF 6V Capacitor: NeoPixels need a capacitor (I used one from Jameco, P/N 606432) to help them run properly.

- 300–500 ohm resistor: NeoPixels also use a resistor. If you don't own any resistors and need to buy them, a good idea is to buy an assortment. The Maker Shed has a nice multipack (P/N MKEE5). Jameco offers a similar assortment (P/N 10720).

- ADXL335 accelerometer: This is a sweet and easy-to-use accelerometer sold by Adafruit (P/N 163). Other online retailers sell similar products featuring the ADXL335 accelerometer chip.

- Male header pins: These pins (SparkFun, P/N 12693) allow you to connect the proto board to your Arduino.

Procedure

Assembly of this project is fairly simple. Follow along with these steps:

1. Insert a row of 15 male header pins into the underside of the proto board and solder them in from the top. You can put the pins into the Arduino if you want to ensure they're straight, as shown in Figure 9-10. One pin will dangle between the analog and power GPIOs—it's the one that looks red in the diagram. All of those Arduino pins will be available to you via the rows of connector holes on the proto board.

2. Solder the accelerometer into the breadboard as shown in Figure 9-11. The sensor comes with header pins that are typically soldered into the accelerometer's PCB; simply solder the other ends into the breadboard.

3. Wire up the accelerometer. Figure 9-12 shows how it should look: the pin marked Xout connects to analog pin A2 on the Arduino, while Yout con-

nects to A1 and Zout to A0. Meanwhile, 5V on the accelerometer (shown as a red wire) connects to the 5V strip and GND plugs into GND via the black wire.

4. Solder in the capacitor. The component is polarized, meaning it has a positive and negative lead. Place the cap as you see in Figure 9-13, then wire the positive lead to the strip plugged into the 5V pin of the Arduino, shown as a cyan wire in the diagram. Next, solder the negative lead into a strip plugged into a ground pin, shown as a purple wire.

5. Next, solder in the resistor as shown in Figure 9-14. Also add a wire (shown in yellow in the diagram) leading from one end of the resistor to digital pin 6 of the Arduino.

6. Solder in the three wires of the LED strand. Figure 9-15 shows an old-style, non-NeoPixel strip with four leads. On the NeoPixel strip there are only three leads: power, ground, and data. Wire them as you see in the figure, with power going from the same row as the positive lead of the capacitor, shown as a cyan wire. The data wire (shown as orange) starts at one end of the resistor and connects to the data pad on the LED strand. Finally, the ground wire (depicted as gray) connects from the negative lead of the capacitor to the GND pad on the strip. You're done!

7. Add the proto board to the Arduino. Simply plug the male headers into the correct pins on the Arduino: all of the power and analog female headers. If the wires leading to the NeoPixel strip are thin enough, they can be trapped between the top and bottom of the Pelican case. Otherwise, you'll have no choice but to drill a hole in the plastic case and its rubber gasket, thread the wires through, then seal up the hole with hot glue.

Installing the Light Strip

You have a couple of options for attaching the light strip to your bike. The strip seems very flexible and rubbery, but it's also fragile. You can't have it flexing around or the solder on the strip will eventually crack. If you're just going to have the strip on temporarily, it would probably be fine to have it coiled around the seat post like you see in Figure 9-16.

However, if you want the strip to be more securely installed, you'll need to zip-tie it to the frame. This presents a problem—how do we get the strip flexing around all the angles of the frame? The solution is to cut apart the strip. Yes, with scissors. On the strip, you'll find little lines with scissors symbols next to them. The lines bisect the big copper solder pads between each LED. Once cut apart, you simply solder on

wires to reconnect them, allowing you to basically decorate your bike however you want. You also have the option of using fewer than 60 LEDs—a strip of 15 on each side of the frame would look great.

One concern you might have is whether the strip can be exposed to the elements. Good news—there is a moisture-resistant plastic sheathing on the NeoPixel strip and you can goop up the ends with hot glue to seal it, allowing you to leave your bike out in the rain. Don't get complacent, however! If there is a tiny crack in the sheathing, you might find yourself with a damaged or destroyed strip.

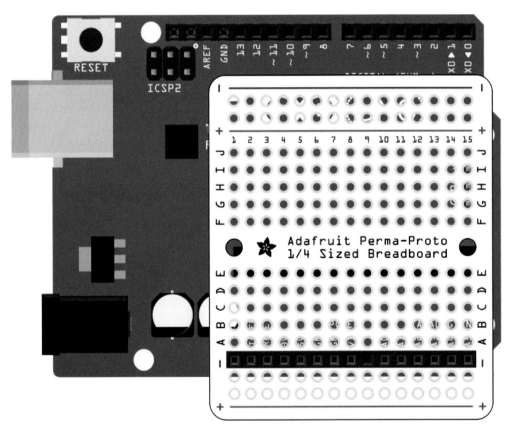

Figure 9-10 *Insert the row of pins into the underside of the board*

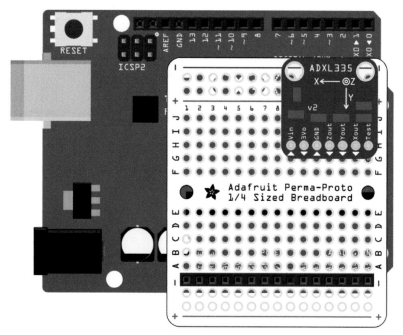

Figure 9-11 *Solder in the accelerometer*

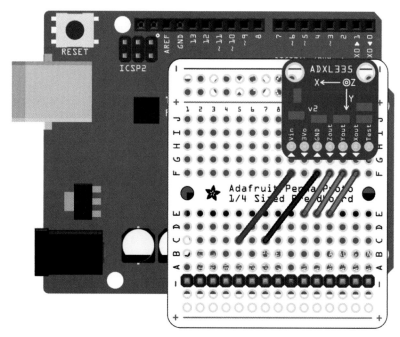

Figure 9-12 *Wire up the accelerometer*

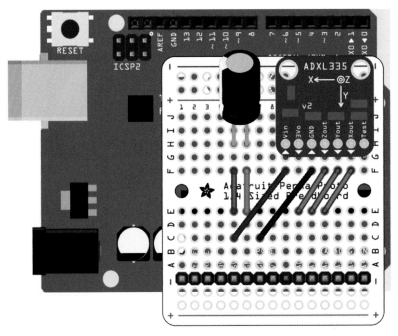

Figure 9-13 *The capacitor gets added next*

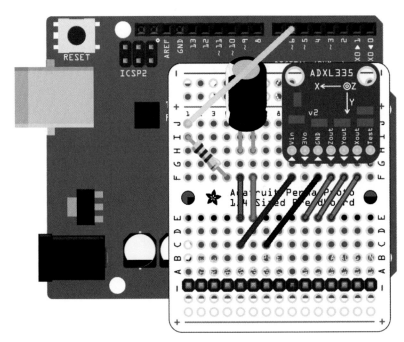

Figure 9-14 *Solder in the resistor*

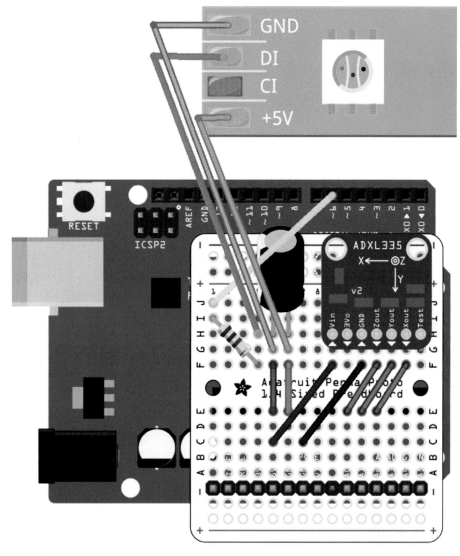

Figure 9-15 *Solder in the wires of the LED strand*

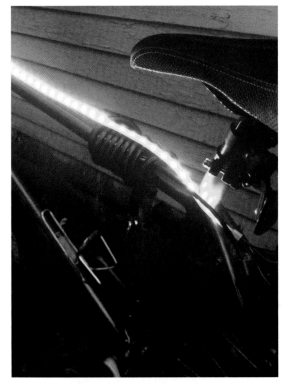

Figure 9-16 *Install the light strip on your bike*

Programming the Arduino

Let's get that Arduino all programmed up. Follow along with these steps:

1. Download the NeoPixel library. Before we even begin to talk about the actual sketch (as Arduino programs are called) let's tackle the NeoPixel library. These are files containing programming functions that are called from the main sketch, keeping the main sketch free of needless code. In order to use the light strip, you'll need to download the Neo-Pixel library (*https://github.com/ adafruit/Adafruit_NeoPixel*). Go to the URL and click the Download Zip button in the righthand column.

2. Rename the folder. The library downloaded with a name that needs to be changed. Rename the NeoPixel library as *Adafruit_NeoPixel*.

3. Put the library in Arduino's *libraries* folder. If you look in the Arduino folder on your computer, you'll find a subdirectory called *libraries*, which contains all the other libraries that came with the Arduino software. Just put the new *Adafruit_NeoPixel* folder alongside those folders.

4. Open up the examples. One of the coolest aspects of libraries is being able to use the example sketches that typically accompany them. Examples are sketches that illustrate the various functions of the libraries. In this case, the NeoPixel sketch is called *strandtest*. You can find examples in the Arduino software under File → Examples. This sketch shows various displays, including wipes and rainbows. However, in my light strip sketch, I used a simple wipe in red just to get you started.

5. Download or type in the sketch detailed in the following section.

The Sketch

Let's take a closer look at the Arduino sketch that controls the light strip. At its heart, the project consists of just two components: the dirt-simple acceleration sensor, which simply returns three analog values for X, Y, and Z, as well as the aforementioned NeoPixel strip. As such, the sketch is fairly simple:

```
/* This sketch makes use of code from David
A. Mellis's ADXL3xx sketch
   and Adafruit's NeoPixel library. */

#include <Adafruit_NeoPixel.h>

/*this pin connects to the light strip's
  data connection */
#define PIN 6

/* accelero input pins */
const int xInput = A0;
const int yInput = A2;
const int zInput = A3;

int idleX = 0;
```

```
int idleY = 0;
int idleZ = 0;

int idlemaxX = 0;
int idlemaxY = 0;
int idlemaxZ = 0;

int idleminX = 0;
int idleminY = 0;
int idleminZ = 0;


/* define light strip */
Adafruit_NeoPixel strip =
                  Adafruit_NeoPixel(60,
PIN, NEO_GRB + NEO_KHZ800);


void setup() {

  Serial.begin(9600); // activate the serial
                      // connection

  pinMode(xInput, INPUT);
  pinMode(yInput, INPUT);
  pinMode(zInput, INPUT);

/* initialize light strip */
  strip.begin();
  strip.show(); /* Initialize all pixels to
'off' */


/* take baseline accelero readings */
  idleX = readAxis(xInput);
  idleY = readAxis(yInput);
  idleZ = readAxis(zInput);

 }

void loop() {

/* take active accelero readings
   not that we need all three axes, right?
All we really need is Y.
   We'll comment out the x and z for now.
*/

/*  int rawX = readAxis(xInput); */
  int rawY = readAxis(yInput);
/*  int rawZ = readAxis(zInput);  */
```

```
/* this computes a number by comparing the
idle with
        the active acceleration  */
int speed= rawY - idleY;

/* comparing the active Y with the idle Y
   if the bike moves forward, the NeoPixels
fire up!  */
      if (rawY > idleY){

        colorWipe(strip.Color(255, 0, 0),
speed); /* wipes in red */
        colorWipe(strip.Color(0, 0, 0),
1); /* wipes out color  */
    }
}


/* function to grab accelerometer data  */

int readAxis(int axisPin)
{
  long reading = 0;
  analogRead(axisPin);
  delay(1);
  for (int i = 0; i < 10; i++)
  {
    reading += analogRead(axisPin);
  }
  return reading/10;
};

/* here's the colorWipe function from the
strandtest example  */

void colorWipe(uint32_t c, uint8_t wait) {
  for(uint16_t i=0; i<strip.numPixels(); i+
+) {
      strip.setPixelColor(i, c);
      strip.show();
      delay(wait);
  }
}
```

Summary

Chapter 9 showed you how to build two cool light-up projects for your bike. Next up, in Chapter 10, you'll tackle a couple of synthesizer projects: a cool musical horn and a motion-sensing alarm.

Making Noise 10

Remember the gentle *ting ting* sound of the classic bike bell from your childhood? Every bike needs a noisemaker, like a horn or bell. It's how you warn pedestrians that you're about to bowl them over. As far as this book is concerned, your bike's noisemaker is yet another thing you can customize. This chapter shows how to make a cool synthesizer horn (Figure 10-1), as well as a motion-sensing bike alarm. Both utilize the same basic method for creating noise: telling the Arduino to send a signal to a speaker.

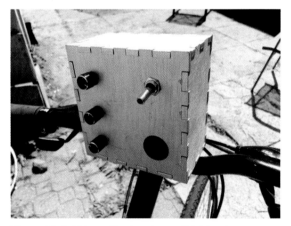

Figure 10-1 *This synthesizer horn will let 'em know you're there*

Audio Synthesizers 101

Back in the first days of integrated circuits (ICs) and microchips, engineers figured out that you could use simple components to make tones that could be played through a speaker. One of the earliest attempts is the now-legendary Stepped Tone Generator (Figure 10-2) created by equally legendary engineer Forrest Mims. The Stepped Tone Generator (which acquired the much cooler moniker Atari Punk Console) is deceptively simple: a timer IC makes a beat, and a second timer IC and a series of potentiometers modifies the beat's speed and pitch. More techniques and components joined the arsenal, adding distortions, reverberations, and other fun audio effects, and electronic music came into its own.

The heart of an analog synth is the tone generator, which creates the beat that forms the underpinning of whatever noise ends up coming out of the speaker. When microcontrollers became commonplace, digital musical synthesis started to replace the analog variety. Putting it bluntly, a computer can make any noise, and hold any beat, while an analog synthesizer is limited to whatever purpose each component was hardwired to perform.

While arguably less fun and cool than an analog synth, digital synths have the advantage of being dirt simple! Most of the work is done in software, allowing you to easily modify the sounds you make without resoldering a thing.

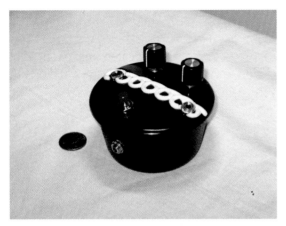

Figure 10-2 *The Atari Punk Console is a classic analog noisemaker (Photo credit: Wayne Wylupski, Community Commons)*

Project #10: Synthesizer, Horn, and Alarm

This chapter's project (Figure 10-3) consists of three parts: a simple buzzer, a synthesizer horn, and an alarm. This project uses an Arduino Uno to generate a waveform, runs that through a small mono amplifier to give it a little zing, and finally pipes it out to a small speaker to create noise. In the synth form, three potentiometers allow you to customize the tune on the fly, or even turn your bike into a mobile synth.

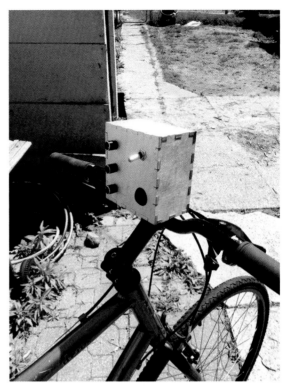

Figure 10-3 *The synthesizer horn will add a new element to your bike*

Parts List

Grab the following parts to build your Synthesizer Horn project:

- A wooden enclosure: I laser-cut my own; you can download the design from Thingiverse (*http://www.thingiverse.com/jwb/*).

- Arduino Uno: Feel free to substitute some other board like an Arduino Pro (SparkFun, P/N 10915) or a Trinket (Adafruit, P/N 1501) in its place.

- Mono 2.5W Amp: This amp is dirt cheap and easy to use! Adafruit (P/N 2130) sells them for only $3.95.

- ADXL335 Accelerometer: You already used this in your NeoPixel strip in Chapter 9 so you probably already know the ADXL335 (Adafruit, P/N 167) is dirt simple to use. You take a reading, and when the module moves, it returns analog signals to show its direction and rate of acceleration.

- Potentiometers (3): I used 10K pots from SparkFun (P/N 9939). It really doesn't matter what rating pots you use. You can also substitute any analog sensor like a light sensor because they all do the same thing: deliver an analog signal to the Arduino. Note that you'll only need these pots if you want to do the synth project.

- Button: I suggest an arcade-style button from SparkFun (P/N 9339).

- Switch: I suggest a simple toggle switch from SparkFun (P/N 9276).

- Keylock switch: This switch (SparkFun, P/N 11473) fits into the same-sized hole as the switch we used already, and serves the same purpose except that it needs a key to turn on and off.

- 4- to 8-ohm speaker: I used one from Adafruit, a 3-watt speaker with 4 ohms of impedence (P/N 1314).

- 10K Resistors (3): You can find some of these in the Maker Shed's resistor assortment (P/N MKEE8).

- Male DC adapter: This adapter (Adafruit, P/N 369) consists of a 2.1mm barrel plug with a pair of terminal blocks on it. This component typically finds use as a power plug for an Arduino or other device powered by a barrel plug.

- Stripboard: This prototyping board (Jameco, P/N 2125042) has rows connected together by copper conductors, and is great for making permanent circuits.

- Wire

Building the Buzzer Horn

Let's start building the noisemaker. To recap: I'm going to show you three flavors of the same general idea (the buzzer horn, the synth, and the bike alarm). Let's begin with the first! The buzzer is so primitive it seems almost blasphemous to use a sophisticated microcontroller like an Arduino Uno on a silly noisemaker, but trust me—the project gets progressively more complicated!

1. Solder up the battery holder and switch (Figure 10-4). The switch is in-line with the power wire of the battery (marked in orange) that plugs into the positive lead of the DC adapter, and the ground wire of the battery plugs into the negative lead of the adapter.

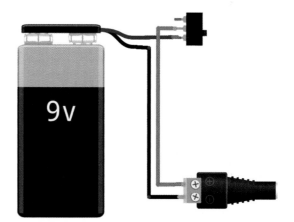

Figure 10-4 *Connect the barrel plug to the battery, with a switch along the way*

2. Connect the Arduino by popping the barrel plug into the appropriate port on the Arduino, shown in Figure 10-5.

3. Next, grab a stripboard and connect two of the rows to power and ground respectively (Figure 10-6). You'll need to solder in the wires on the board end, but can get away with just sliding the wire-ends into the Arduino's female headers. Note that stripboard can be cut apart with a hacksaw if it's too big.

4. Wire in the button. This is somewhat complicated as it includes a resistor. One lead of the button (a pink wire in Figure 10-7) solders into a row of the stripboard. The same row gets a wire leading to pin 2 of the Arduino (orange in the figure). The row also gets the 10K resistor soldered in, leading to a different row. That row connects to ground via a soldered wire (purple). Finally, the other lead of the button connects to ground via a wire (brown) soldered into place.

5. Connect the amp (see Figure 10-8). The amp has five holes you can solder wires or pins into. A+ is the audio source (in this case, digital pin 8 on the Arduino), which first gets soldered into the breadboard (shown as yellow wire) and

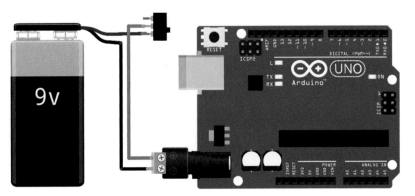

Figure 10-5 *Add the Arduino*

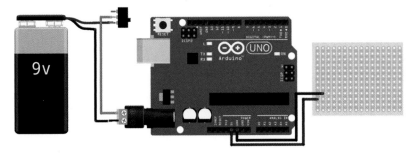

Figure 10-6 *Connect the stripboard*

from there to the amp (red wire). The pin marked A- plugs into ground (shown as a black wire). VIN and GND are power (green wire) and ground (gray), respectively, for the amp, and these solder into the stripboard's power and ground rows. Finally, plug the speaker's leads into the screw terminals on the amp. You're done!

Programming the buzzer horn

For the horn, start with one of the example sketches that you downloaded along with the Arduino software called toneMelody, in the Arduino IDE menu under File→Examples→Digital. toneMelody plays a song when your Arduino powers up. I'll show you how to modify the sketch to make a rude buzz (for those joyless souls who don't want music) or to change the tune so it's something you like better. After that I'll show you how to make the horn into a simple synth that makes cool noises when you fiddle with the potentiometers!

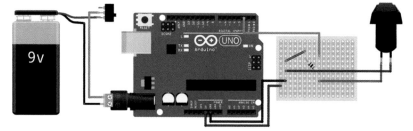

Figure 10-7 *Connect the button and its resistor*

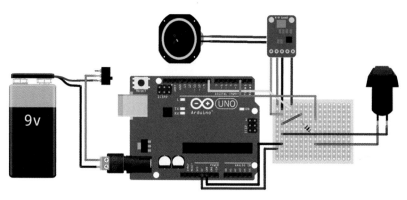

Figure 10-8 *Connect the amp*

Let's get started with the first sketch:

```
/*Synthesizer Horn */
/*Based off the toneMelody example sketch
by Tom Igoe. */

#include "pitches.h"
/*these are the preprogrammed pitches
  (notes) that the sketch plays. The
  nomenclature is the note letter and
  octave, so G3 is the "G" note one
  octave above G2. I'm just alternating
  the two notes very quickly.  */

const int buttonPin = 2;
int buttonState = 0;
int thisNote;
int noteDuration;

/*the following array consists of the tune
to be played.
  You can make it as long or short as you
want,
  but be sure to change the noteDurations[]
array and the
  number of tones in the melody (currently
8) in the loop.  */

int melody[] = {
  NOTE_G2, NOTE_G3, NOTE_G2, NOTE_G3,
NOTE_G2,
  NOTE_G3, NOTE_G2, NOTE_G3};

/* an array of note durations corresponding
to each note;
  4 = quarter note, 8 = eighth note, etc.
*/

int noteDurations[] = {
  4,4,4,4,4,4,4,4};

void setup() {

  pinMode(buttonPin, INPUT);

}


void loop() {


  /* listen for the button  */
  buttonState = digitalRead(buttonPin);

  int noteDuration = 1000/noteDurations[this
Note];
```

```
  if (buttonState == HIGH) {
    /* play the tune */

    for (int thisNote = 0; thisNote < 8;
thisNote++) {
      tone(8, melody[thisNote],noteDura
tion);
      delay(100);
      noTone(8);
      delay(10); /* time between notes,
      measured in milliseconds  */
    }
  }
  else {
    noTone(8);
  }


}
```

Adding a melody in place of the buzz

OK, so how do we get rid of that annoying siren and put in something more dynamic? It probably goes without saying that you'll need to adjust the array that has all the notes in it, the array of note durations, as well as the number of total notes in the loop, so that they reflect the sound you want.

If you need help composing music, you can often find songs in musical notation on the Web. Typically these are simple tunes meant for recorders and tin whistles. You'll have to adjust the durations manually, but they can give you the notes. I should warn you ahead of time that whatever tune you come up with is likely not to be very pleasing to the ear—only slightly more so than the siren!

If you want to learn more about Arduino's Tone sketches, see their reference page (*http://ardui no.cc/en/reference/tone*).

Building the Synth

By synth, I mean a noisemaker like the horn, but whose tempo, pitch, and note duration are controlled manually with the help of potentiometers, letting you fiddle with the knobs to make weird noises. In addition to the pots, you'll be adding a switch that is wired up in parallel with the button, and accomplishing the same thing (turning on the noise) with the obvious exception that it stays on or off. Here are the steps you'll need to follow:

1. Install the pots. Figure 10-9 shows how to do it: the middle lead of each pot (marked with orange wires) goes to pins A3-5 on the Arduino. The side pins are 5V and GND, marked with red and black wires, respectively.

2. Add the switch in parallel with the button (Figure 10-10).

3. Reprogram the Arduino. This is a simple sketch that nevertheless lets you make some cool noises! It's based on the Arduino example sketch tonePitch-Follower, which controls the pitch (the sound it makes) with the help of an analog sensor. Our sketch will be a little more sophisticated, also controlling the duration of the notes as well as the amount of time between notes. At the same time, it still allows you to press the button to buzz someone—it will just be the synth playing when you do.

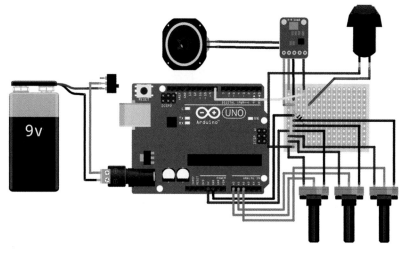

Figure 10-9 *Solder in the potentiometers*

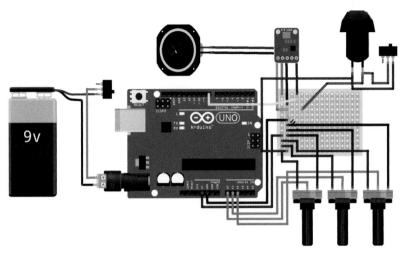

Figure 10-10 *The switch gets wired in parallel to the button*

Here's the code for the sketch:

```
/*Based on the example sketch
tonePitchFollower by Tom Igoe. */

int pitchPot = A0;
int durationPot = A1;
int delayPot = A2;

void setup() {
}

void loop() {

  int pitchReading = analogRead(A0);
  int durationReading = analogRead(A1);
  int delayReading = analogRead(A2);

/* ok, let's translate the range of the
pots (0 to 1023) into the range we need for
the various controls. For instance, pitch
ranges from 120 through 1500 Hz so our read
ing from the pot has to be converted. */

  int thisPitch = map(pitchReading, 0,
1023, 120, 1500);

/* now let's do duration, which is how long
each tone lasts. I don't want each tone to
exceed half-a-second in length, so the
range is 10 to 500 milliseconds. */

int thisDuration = map(durationReading, 0,
1023, 10, 500);

/* duplicate these values for the delay:  */
```

```
int thisDelay = map(delayReading, 0, 1023,
10, 500);

/* so here is the meat of the sketch: */

  tone(8, thisPitch, thisDuration);
  delay(thisDelay);
}
```

Bicycle Alarm

The alarm is simply the horn project triggered by an accelerometer if the bike is moved without the keylock switch being turned. Best of all, you can even have the synth functionality unchanged; the accelerometer plugs into free ports on the Arduino. You will, however, have to reprogram the Arduino to accommodate the new hardware.

Procedure

The following steps assume you have built the horn and synth project, so make sure you complete that project before moving ahead. Here's what you'll need to do:

1. Add the accelerometer. You're already familiar with the ADXL335. It has power and ground connectors, and three data

leads that plug into analog ports. You can see how to wire it up in Figure 10-11: Z plugs into A0, Y into 1, and Z into 2. You can connect the power and ground to the proper rows on the stripboard using short wires.

2. Add the keylock switch. When turned on, the switch tells the sketch to pay attention to the accelerometer and to buzz if the bike is moved. Figure 10-12 shows one of these switches.

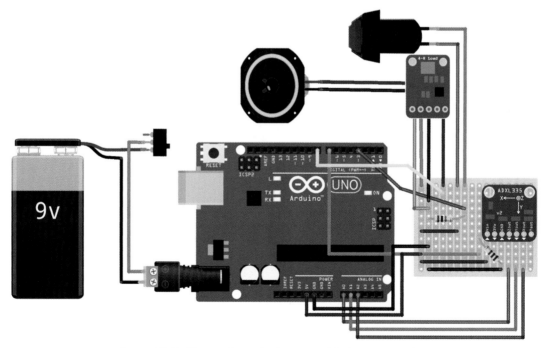

Figure 10-11 *The accelerometer turns your bike horn into an alarm*

Code

The sketch is remarkably similar to the horn sketch, with the accelerometer replacing the button as the triggering mechanism. Additionally, the horn continues for two minutes before turning off.

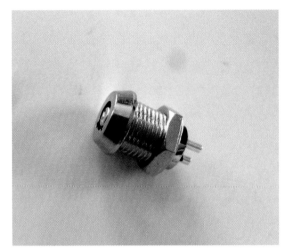

Figure 10-12 *The keylock switch works the same as a regular switch, as long as you have the key!*

```
/* Bike alarm
     Based off the toneMelody example sketch
by Tom Igoe.   */

#include "pitches.h"

/* accelerometer inputs */

const int xInput = A5;
const int yInput = A4;
const int zInput = A3;

int idleX = 0; int idleY = 0; int idleZ = 0;
int idlemaxX = 0; int idlemaxY = 0; int idle
maxZ = 0;
int idleminX = 0; int idleminY = 0; int idle
minZ = 0;


void setup() {

  pinMode(xInput, INPUT);
  pinMode(yInput, INPUT);
  pinMode(zInput, INPUT);

  /* baseline readings for the
     accelerometer */
```

```
  idleX = readAxis(xInput);
  idleY = readAxis(yInput);
  idleZ = readAxis(zInput);

}


void loop() {

 /* read current accelerometer data   */

  int rawX = readAxis(xInput);
  int rawY = readAxis(yInput);
  int rawZ = readAxis(zInput);


   /* next, a statement that detects whether
the bike has been moved
        by comparing the idle G-force with the
current G-force.
        If the bike moves even an inch, plug
your ears!   */

  if(rawX>idleX||rawX>idleX||rawX>idleX){

 /* pin 8, 554 hertz, lasting for 120,000
  milliseconds   */
  tone(8,554,120000);

delay(10);
  }

  else {
    noTone(8);
  }


}
/* function to grab accelerometer data   */

int readAxis(int axisPin)
{
  long reading = 0;
  analogRead(axisPin);
  delay(1);
  for (int i = 0; i < 10; i++)
  {
    reading += analogRead(axisPin);
  }
  return reading/10;
}
```

Summary

We went all audio in this chapter, adding lovely sound to our bikes in the form of a digital synthesizer horn that beeps or plays a simple tune when you press a button. You further enhanced the project with a keylock switch and an accelerometer so it serves as an alarm against anyone messing with your bike. Next up, in Chapter 11, you'll learn two ways to carry stuff on your bike.

Hauling Cargo 11

One of the greatest challenges of bike riding since its inception has been how to also carry stuff. A bike can transport a cyclist perfectly well. But that rider and his or her groceries—that's another matter. Motorists take for granted how easy it is to haul cargo in a car. Heck, most of the time you can just throw whatever you're carrying onto a seat.

Bikes are handicapped by not having a horizontal surface as standard equipment. The inherent instability of bicycles doesn't help either. There are options, of course. For instance, cargo bikes are big, heavy bikes, usually with a wooden platform incorporated into the frame. These bikes are a lifesaver if you've got groceries, but what if you're just tooling around the neighborhood? Riding around in such a bike would get a little old. There is a lot of middle ground between a cargo bike and nothing at all. In this chapter, you'll learn about some common cargo-carrying options in the cycling world. Then I'll guide you through creating two kinds of carriers: a basket (seen in Figure 11-1) and a small trailer.

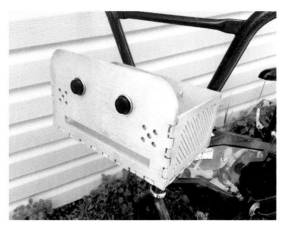

Figure 11-1 *I'll show you how to build this fun basket*

Typical Cargo-Hauling Options

The following are typical cargo-hauling options found in bike stores everywhere.

Basket

We most often associate bike baskets with kids' bikes or those used by delivery riders. It's a convenient and low-maintenance way to haul small objects around. Furthermore, if it's the sort of basket mounted on the front handlebars, it becomes the focal point and a great opportunity to spiff up your bike with a pretty one.

Panniers

Classic saddlebags, panniers are good for hauling moderate amounts of cargo. It is possible to get a pair of panniers each able to carry a standard grocery bag, though most of the time they're smaller. Panniers often come in pairs, usually mounted to either side of the back wheels (though they can sometimes be mounted to the front wheels). In an ideal world, you'll want to balance the weight contained in each pack, though you can still ride with an unbalanced load.

Rack

The ultimate in customizable storage space, racks serve as a horizontal space with bungee mounting points. These allow you to carry a variety of things like bags and boxes, but also don't take up a lot of room. They're lightweight, low-maintenance, and inexpensive. On the downside, racks lack the ability to hold small or un-bungee-able things, the way a basket could.

Trailer

Like a freight bike with a removable cargo unit, a trailer holds a bunch of stuff but can itself be stored away when not needed. Like anything relating to bicycles, it's better for a trailer to be as light as possible.

Project #11: Bike Basket Project

Let's begin with a simple bike project: building your own basket (Figure 11-2). OK, it's more of a box, laser-cut out of plywood and mounted on your handlebars, but it holds stuff and that's what you need. Just to make it more fun, I designed mine to look like a robot using reflectors for the eyes.

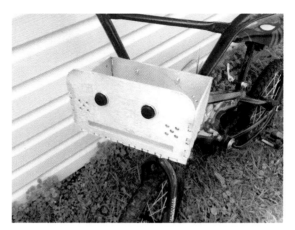

Figure 11-2 *This robot basket will rock a bike!*

Parts List

You'll need the following parts to build your basket:

- Wood basket parts: These should be laser- or hand-cut out of quarter-inch medium-density fiberboard (MDF) or plywood. My design is on Thingiverse (*http://www.thingiverse.com/jwb*).

- 3D-printed bike clamps: I printed out a couple of Cameron Stewart's bike mounts and they work great in conjunction with a rubber band for friction. You can find these mounts on Thingiverse (*http://www.thingiverse.com/thing:37328*). If you don't have access to a 3D printer, I suggest looking online for a bicycle mount kit, or repurpose another bike accessory's mounting hardware. Finally, you may be able to simply zip-tie the basket in place.

- Wood glue

- Spray paint

- Reflectors: I found some 1" reflectors with a wingnut connector at a thrift store. I can't give you a part number, but I found similar ones online after searching for "license plate reflector bolts."

Procedure

Now, it's time to put the parts together and build your basket:

1. Decide what shape you want your basket to be: small and compact or big and capacious? As mentioned, I've included a design on my Thingiverse page, but feel free to create your own! The main thing to remember is that a small basket may be supported by just the handlebars (Figure 11-3) but a big one will need to be supported some other way, such as by stays connected to an axle or otherwise bolted to the frame. I'll explain how to do that at the end of the basket build.

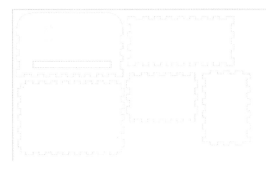

Figure 11-4 *The laser follows this pattern to cut out the parts*

3. Use wood glue to assemble the parts of the basket, as seen in Figure 11-5.

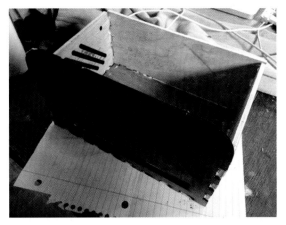

Figure 11-5 *Assemble the basket, gluing the seams with regular wood glue*

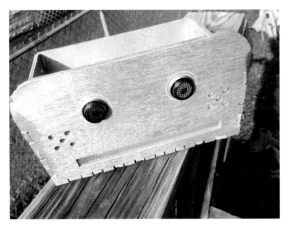

Figure 11-3 *This basket is just the thing to robot up your bike*

2. Laser or mill out the design using quarter-inch plywood or MDF. You can see the pattern from my project in Figure 11-4.

4. Paint the basket. This isn't just to make it look pretty—the paint will help protect the basket from the elements. You can see how my basket turned out in Figure 11-6.

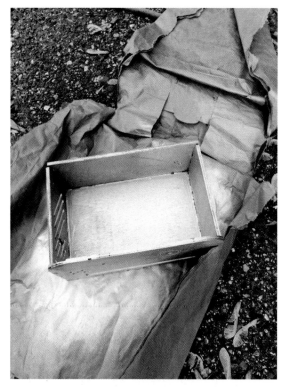

Figure 11-6 *A couple coats of spray paint will make the basket last longer*

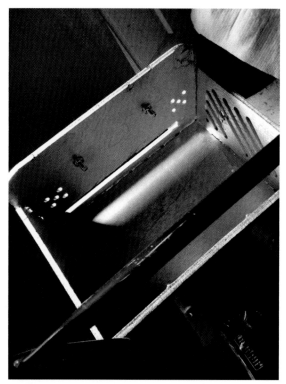

Figure 11-7 *Reflectors add visibility and look awesome*

5. Add reflectors to the front of the basket, as seen in Figure 11-7. It doesn't hurt to add a little visibility, and you might as well make it cute!

6. Attach the tube clamps or 3D-printed handlebar mounts to the connector bar using #6-32 socket head screws. Figure 11-8 shows how it should look.

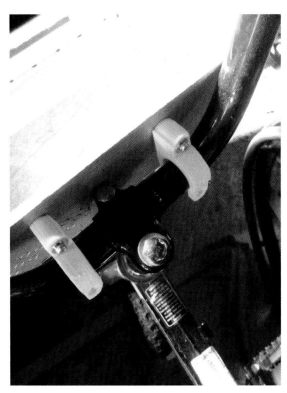

Figure 11-8 *Mount the basket to the handbars*

Make front axle supports

This is a simple way to give your basket extra support, by connecting it to the front axle with the help of metal stays. Here's what you'll need to do:

1. Cut out two lengths of flat metal stock, 12 gauge by a half-inch across.

2. Drill holes in either end: the axle end's hole should have a diameter compatible with the axle, while the basket side should have 3/16th-inch holes drilled into them.

3. Bend the stays so they extend from the basket to the axle.

4. Attach the stays to the axle, using the normal hex nuts used to secure the wheel.

5. Attach the stays to the basket, using #8-32 screws, nuts, and washers.

As an alternative, you can often find axle supports on baskets, child seats, and other bicycle accessories (check your local thrift store), and these can be put to use for your project.

Project #12: Mini Trailer

This mini trailer (Figure 11-9) was created by re-purposing an old wheelchair.

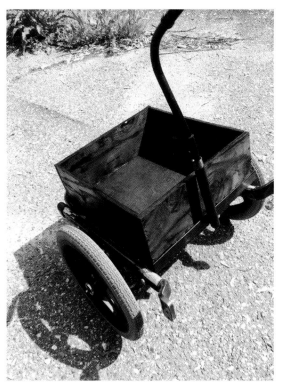

Figure 11-9 *The mini trailer is made to haul modest loads of cargo*

This chair was my dad's, and wasn't safe to be used anymore. Rather than consigning it to a landfill, I decided to part it out. I was mostly looking at the big wheels, as they were already mounted on sturdy 8mm shafts with handy bolt-on mounts ready to go. However, once I got the wheels off, I realized that the frame itself would make a great platform, and already had the mounting holes for the wheels! I figured I'd remount the wheels in the middle of the structure and weld the hardware for a cargo platform directly to the frame. Don't worry, however—if you don't have a wheelchair to use, I'll show you how to build the trailer without one.

Parts List

In order to build your trailer, you'll need the following parts:

- Angle iron: I just used some scrap angle iron. This is commonplace metal extruded at an angle. The classic example is the metal used to make a bed frame.

- Wheelchair frame: This metal frame is pierced with 8mm holes to accommodate wheel mounts.

- Wheels: You can get any number of great wheels. I suggest either bicycle wheels or lawnmower wheels from Harbor Freight or a similar store.

- Axle: The wheel assemblies I harvested each have their own small axle—rather than sharing a common one. Get an axle to match your wheels.

- Towbar: How will you tow the trailer? You'll need to buy or make a bar that connects the bike to the trailer.

- Half-inch plywood: You'll need one 18"×18" and four 6"×18" pieces.

- Spray paint

- Wood screws: A bunch of #6 × 1"

Procedure

Follow these steps to build your mini trailer:

1. Cut the four 18" lengths of angle iron, as shown in Figure 11-10. You should choose the lengths based on how big a cargo bed you want. I chose those lengths because the angle iron I found was only so long (part of the fun of lengths, as shown in Figure 11-10), and because I ultimately want the ability to

haul a cooler around. The cooler I have in mind has a base 17" × 20"—I'm adding extra space for the trailer's walls.

If you want to get elite, cut each end at a 45° angle to facilitate arranging them as a rectangle.

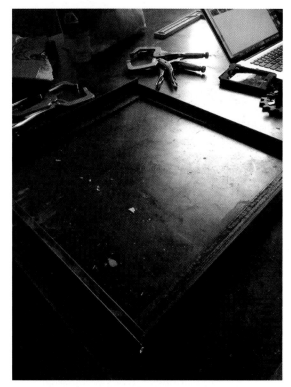

Figure 11-10 *Cut lengths of angle iron in order to build your bed*

2. Weld or braze the angle iron together. Use the skills you developed in Chapter 7 to attach the parts together. As shown in Figure 11-11, the parts are arranged horizontally and then welded up. I chose to make them 6 inches, just cuz.

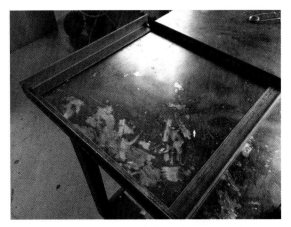

Figure 11-11 *Weld or braze the trailer's frame*

3. Attach the angle iron to the wheelchair frame, either by welding it or bolting it on. If you're not using a wheelchair, now is the time to get creative. Here are a couple of options:

   - Simply weld kiddie bike forks to the frame, effectively giving you ready-to-go wheels. Just make sure you have the forks pointing in the same direction!

   - Use ordinary bike dropouts, as in Figure 11-12, that can be welded to the frame.

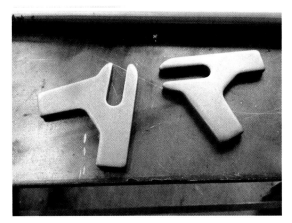

Figure 11-12 *Weld on the dropouts*

4. Add the towbar attachment. The towbar is the bar that pulls the trailer be-

hind it. You could weld up your own, but I'm suggesting a standard bike towbar, found in any bicycle store. The typical configuration serves to attach a child's bike to the parent's, and consists of a bar with a loop on each end—one loop passes around the parent's seat tube and the other loop around the kid's head tube.

Cut a 7–9" length of 1-inch pipe (seen on the left in Figure 11-13) and weld it on vertically. The towbar should happily hold on to this vertical tube. You can add a cap to the threaded end if the towbar slips off.

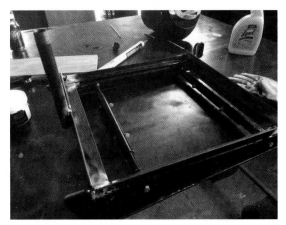

Figure 11-13 *This tube helps pull the trailer behind the bike*

5. Begin building the cargo box. I started with an 18" × 18" panel of half-inch plywood, then added walls of a similar material. I cut the walls 6" high, because I wanted a low profile on the trailer. Begin by gluing and clamping one of the walls (Figure 11-13) and then secure it with #6 x 1" screws, making sure to predrill the holes.

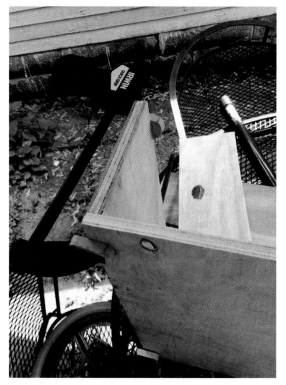

Figure 11-14 *Begin making the cargo box out of plywood*

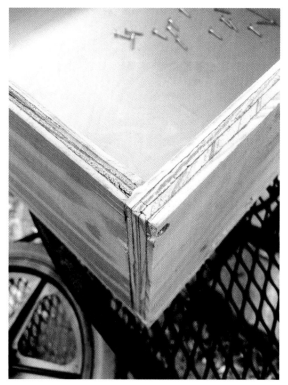

Figure 11-15 *Attach the second and third walls*

6. Add the second and third walls. You may need to trim two of the 6″ x 18″ boards so that they fit inside the gap of the other two, as shown in Figure 11-15.

7. Attach the final wall, seen in Figure 11-16. Double-check that all the boards are connected to each other.

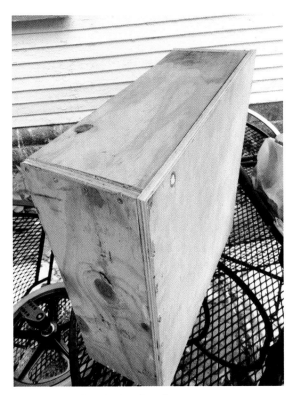

Figure 11-16 *Add the fourth wall*

8. Spray-paint the trailer. Definitely hit all iron and wood components so they don't decay if the trailer is left out in

the rain. Figure 11-17 shows my trailer finished.

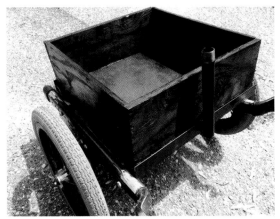

Figure 11-17 *Paint the trailer to protect it from the elements*

Summary

In Chapter 11, we delved into the topic of hauling cargo with your bike. You made a handle-bar-mounted bike basket as well as a mini trailer. In Chapter 12, you'll dress the trailer up with a cooler, light show, and speaker set.

Party Trailer

This is the final chapter in the book! The party trailer project featured in this chapter represents the culmination of a couple different projects that were featured earlier in the book. The trailer, which you just completed, forms the backbone of this project. The "party" comes in with an LED-strand light organ that changes its color and pattern based on the environment around it. We'll use the same NeoPixel light strip that we used in Chapter 9.

Projet #13: Light Organ

The party trailer's light organ consists of an Arduino with a mic hooked up to it, which translates audio levels into lights. It responds to the music by increasing the number of LEDs lit up as well as their color. The Arduino simply uses math to figure out the average low, midrange, and high audio levels, translating that into lit-up LEDs.

Adding to the fun is the presence of a temperature and humidity sensor, allowing us to further alter the light display by having it respond to those factors as well.

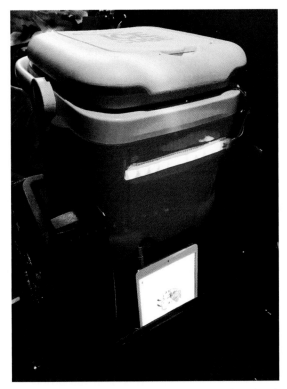

Figure 12-1 *The party trailer brings light, sound, and cool beverages to the party*

Parts List

You'll need the following parts to build the party trailer's light organ:

- Arduino Uno

- AM2302 temperature and humidity sensor (Adafruit, P/N 393): It's functionally identical to the DHT-22 but has wired pins and a different plastic housing.

- Electret Microphone Breakout (SparkFun, P/N 9964): This handy board has a mini microphone along with an op-amp to boost the signal.

- Adafruit NeoPixel Digital RGB LED Strip (P/N 1461)

- 220-ohm resistor

- 1,000uF capacitor

- Adafruit Perma-Proto board (half-size, P/N 571)

- Male header pins (SparkFun, P/N 12693)

Procedure

Let's solder up the proto board with the various components that make up the light organ:

1. Insert male header pins, corresponding to the Arduino's power and analog pins 8 and 6, into the photo board from the underside, as seen in Figure 12-2. Solder them into place from the top of the board. This board will end up connected to the Arduino, and the microcontroller's pins will break out to the rows on the board.

2. Solder in wires leading from the 5V (the orange wire in Figure 12-3) and GND (purple wire) pins of the Arduino to the power and ground buses on the other side of the board.

3. Plug in the microphone module. This small board has three pinouts, and I'm assuming you're going to solder it directly into the proto board. However, if your Arduino is far away from the music, you might want to position the mic closer and run long wires back to the microcontroller. Following along with Figure 12-4 you can see that the power wire (red in the figure) goes into the power bus, and the GND (black) into the GND bus; the data pin connects to Analog 0 using the green wire.

4. Next, add the temperature sensor. The power and ground wires connect as expected to the buses on the proto board, as shown in Figure 12-5. The data wire (the yellow wire in the figure) can be soldered into the proto board rather than plugging it straight into the Arduino. A wire that moves around a lot is likely to fall out of the Arduino header.

5. Lastly, wire in the light strip. The Adafruit NeoPixel strip I used only has three pins, unlike the ones shown in Figure 12-6, but Fritzing (the circuit diagram program I use) lacks the 3-pin light strips in its library. So imagine the yellow wires connect the various strips together through their applicable data-in or data-out pins.

Connect the data wire of the LED strip to pin 6 of the Arduino with a 220-ohm resistor in between. I show the data wire in yellow from the strip to the proto board, then the resistor connecting to another row, where a gray wire connects to pin 6.

The power and ground work as you would imagine except for one key point: a 1000uF capacitor is soldered across the power and ground leads. You can see in the figure that short wires bring in 5V and GND from the buses, the red and black wires from the LED strip connect to the same rows, and the capacitor is soldered in as well.

The last thing I want to mention about the LED strip is that you can cut it into pieces, and simply wire the pieces together: ground to ground, 5V to 5V, data to data, as shown in Figure 12-6.

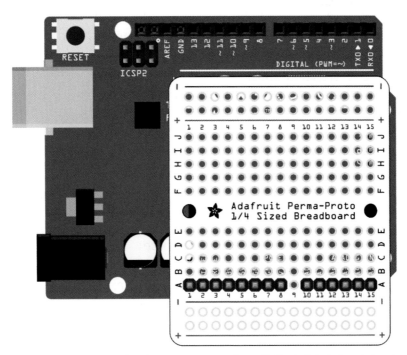

Figure 12-2 *Insert male header pins corresponding with the Arduino's female headers*

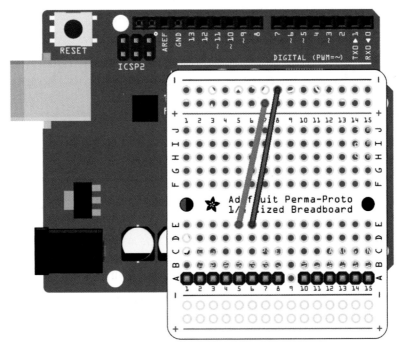

Figure 12-3 *Solder in power and ground wires*

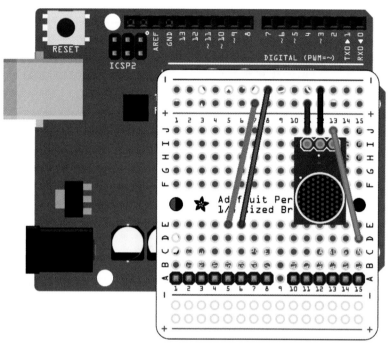

Figure 12-4 *Attach the microphone module*

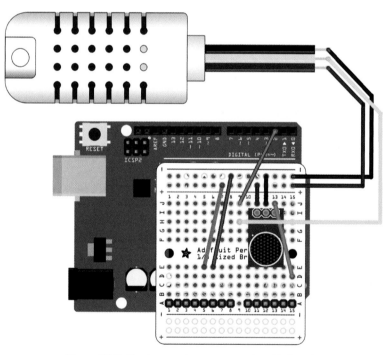

Figure 12-5 *The temperature sensor gets added next*

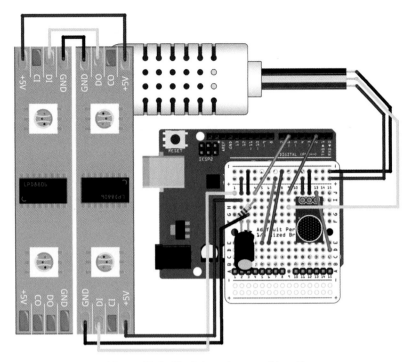

Figure 12-6 *The light strips get soldered in*

Programming the Light Organ

The light organ's sketch consists of a NeoPixel-controlling function and a series of sensor readings that take in the low, middle, and high tones of the music, as well as the ambient temperature, and change the color of the LEDs accordingly. You can download the DHT (temperature sensor) and NeoPixel libraries from Git-Hub (*https://github.com/adafruit/*). Here is the code you'll need:

```
#include <Adafruit_NeoPixel.h>
#include <DHT.h>

#define PIN 6
#define DHTPIN 2

#define DHTTYPE DHT22    // DHT 22  (AM2302)
// specifies which model of temp sensor

int mic_pin = A0;

Adafruit_NeoPixel strip = Adafruit_NeoPix
el(60, PIN, NEO_GRB + NEO_KHZ800);
```

```
void setup() {

  strip.begin();
  strip.show(); // Initialize all pixels
              // to 'off'
  Serial.begin(9600);

  pinMode(mic_pin, INPUT);

}

void loop() {

// listens to mic

int raw_sound = analogRead(sensorPin);

// measures low sounds
int low_sound = raw_sound / 4;
redLight = map(low_sound, 0, 255, 0, 255);

//measures mid sounds
int mid_sound = raw_sound / 2;
greenLight = map(mid_sound, 0, 511, 0, 255);

//measures high sounds
blueLight = map (raw_sound, 0, 1027, 0,
255);
```

```
// listens to temperature sensor
// the sensor can also sense humidity,
// but I didn't do anything with that
// capability; see the DHT library for
// info on how to do this.

   float raw_temp = dht.readTempera
ture(true);

// widget turns temperature into 0-100
int adj_temp = map(raw_temp, 50, 100, 0,
100);

// this colors the pixels according to
// the low, midrange, and high tones.
colorWipe(strip.Color(redLight, greenLight,
blueLight), adj_temp);

}

// this is the function that colors all of
```

```
// the pixels.
void colorWipe(uint32_t c, uint8_t wait) {
  for(uint16_t i=0; i<strip.numPixels(); i+
+) {
      strip.setPixelColor(i, c);
      strip.show();
      delay(wait);
   }
}
```

Summary

Make: Bicycle Projects has come to an end. Now it's time to put your new knowledge to use by hacking on your favorite (or least favorite) bike! Whether it's decorating your bike, hacking its frame, or adding an electronic widget, hopefully this book has you primed to explore the myriad of options for making your bike work better for you.

Index

About the Author

John Baichtal has written or edited over a dozen books, including the award-winning *Cult of Lego* (No Starch Press), *LEGO Hacker Bible*, *Make: LEGO and Arduino Projects* with Adam Wolf and Matthew Beckler (Maker Media), *Robot Builder* (Que), and *Basic Robot Building with LEGO Mindstorms NXT 2.0* (Que), as well as *Building Your Own Drones* (forthcoming from Que). His most recent book is *Maker Pro* (Maker Media), a collection of essays and interviews describing life as a professional maker. John lives in Minneapolis with his wife and three children.